Acta Neurochirurgica
Supplements

Editor: H.-J. Reulen
Assistant Editor: H.-J. Steiger

Advances in Epilepsy Surgery and Radiosurgery

Edited by
B. Sutter and O. Schröttner

Acta Neurochirurgica
Supplement 84

Springer-Verlag Wien GmbH

B. Sutter
O. Schröttner
Universitätsklinik für Neurochirurgie, Karl-Franzens Universität, Graz, Austria

Typesetting: Asco Typesetters, Hong Kong
SPIN: 10883840

With 22 partly coloured Figures

CIP Data applied for

ISSN 0065-1419

ISBN 3-211-83837-6 Springer-Verlag Wien New York

Preface

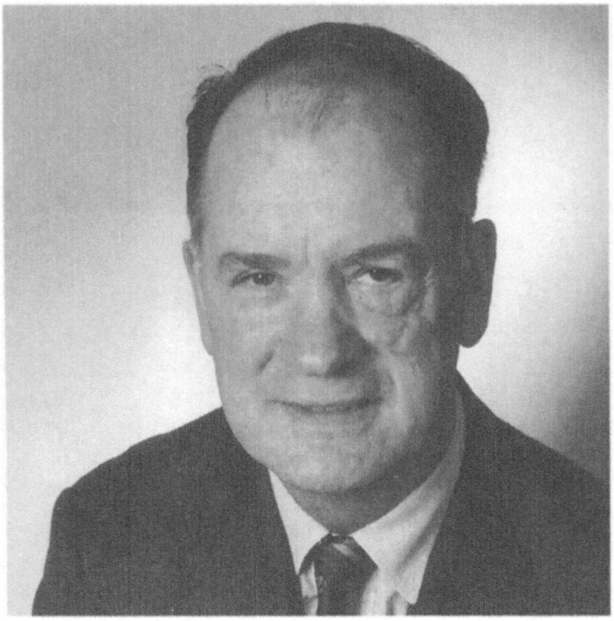

On September 30th, 2002 Professor Gerhard Pendl, M.D. retires from his chairmanship at the Department of Neurosurgery at the University Hospital in Graz.

Shortly after his birth on July 10, 1934 in Linz the family moved to Germany. In 1938 the Pendl family came back to Linz where he spent the rest of his childhood. Finishing school in 1949 he started as a pharmacist and continued till 1957. During his time as a pharmacist he went back to school and graduated on February 22, 1957. Shortly afterwards he started studying medicine at the University of Vienna Medical School. Despite a lot of activities like in his fraternity or as an elected representative of the students' parlament, he graduated in June 1964 as Medical Doctor. In August 1964 he started his medical career in his home town Linz. In 1965 he moved back to Vienna, where he served till 1972 at the new established neurosurgical department under Professor Kraus. During all that time there were a lot of activities: in 1966 and 1967 fellow at the Department of Neurosurgery, Professor James Watts at the George Washington University in Washington D.C., and at the Columbia University New York. In 1967 and 1968 he worked as a general surgeon at the 1st Surgical Department of the Vienna Medical School with Professor Fuchsig. At the Max-Planck Institute in Munich he worked in the years 1968 to 1969 as a neuropathologist. In the year 1969 till 1972 back at the Department of Neurosurgery in Vienna he served as a general neurosurgeon and one of his main goals was pediatric neurosurgery. In August 1972 he moved to Kiel to work with Professor Jensen at the Neurosurgical University Hospital. He had to graduate one more time in Germany and he did this with "Ultrasound Tomography in Neurosurgery". Together with the Department of Pediatrics he started to build the Pediatric Neurosurgical Department. At this time he started his research on pineal, midbrain and brainstem surgery. In September 1976 he started at the Ostsee Clinic Damp in Schleswig-Holstein to build a Neurosurgical Department that opened its gates on 1977 and he became the first chairman. On April 1, 1978 he went back to Vienna as the Vice Chairman of the Department of Neurosurgery at the University Hospital in Vienna under Professor Koos and in 1980 he got his Ph.D. for his work "Microtopographic Operative Ways to the Midbrain and Pineal Region". His most interests were brainstem surgery, epilepsy surgery, pediatric neurosurgery and neurooncology. In 1990 he became Chairman and Professor at the Department of Neurosurgery at the University of Graz Medical School. He started planning and building a new neurosurgical department rebuilding the ICU and the ORs. In 1992 he established the first Austrian Gamma Knife and furtheron one of his main interest was the research in radiosurgery. His most interest was in functional radiosurgery for Parkinson, epilepsy and pain.

Since 1992 he also served in the Medical Faculty as a Vice Dean and in October 1997 till 1999 he became Dean of the University of Graz Medical Faculty. Without rest since then he was thought to achieve dynamic development and his work is dedicated to the constant search for perfection in neurosurgery. His friends and colleagues wish Professor Gerhard Pendl all the best in his retirement and dedicate this issue of Acta Neurochirurgica to him.

Acknowledgment

I gratefully acknowledge manuscript preparation by Mrs Elfriede Meier and expert technical assistance by Mrs Silvia Schilgerius, Springer Verlag. The publisher thanks all the authors for delivering their manuscript in time and Professor Hans-Jürgen Reulen enabling the publication as the responsible chief-editor for Acta Neurochirurgica. This book was made possible by financial support from numerous companies.

Bernhard Sutter, M.D.
Department of Neurosurgery
University of Graz Medical School
Austria

Contents

Listed in Current Contents

Acta Neurochir (2002) [Suppl] 84: 1–16

Future Aspects of Epilepsy Research

H. G. Wieser

Neurology Clinic, Dept. Epileptology and Electroencephalography, University Hospital, Zurich, Switzerland

Summary

This contribution in honour of Prof. Gerhard Pendl first reviews some recent studies on resected tissue, migrational disorders, and Rasmussen's Syndrome. These areas of basic research profit from recent advances of molecular biology and genetics. On the clinical side, some studies dealing with proton magnetic resonance spectroscopy are reviewed. In order to highlight the progress in clinical epilepsy research using modern methods of structural and functional imaging, functional outcome prediction is also reviewed. This kind of advanced clinical research is dealt with by discussing risk factor assessment associated with postsurgical decrements in memory. With regard to motor functions, we compare the yield of functional MR and intraoperative cortical stimulation in patients with lesions in or close to the Rolandic cortex. Progress in the field of advanced EEG analysis is reviewed in the context of "seizure prediction" and cognitive event-related potentials. Finally some of the new epilepsy treatment options, such as Gamma Knife treatment, where Prof. Pendl's group made pioneering contributions, are dealt with.

Keywords: Experimental and clinical epilepsy research; epilepsy surgery.

Introduction

Given the title of my contribution I decided that I should start my review with basic research in resected tissue, migrational disorders, and Rasmussen's Syndrome. This type of research substantially profits from recent advances of molecular biology and genetics. On the clinical side proton magnetic resonance spectroscopy (1H-MRS) offers to study non-invasively some elementary processes involved in epileptogenesis. In the daily clinical work, prediction of functional outcome after surgery becomes increasingly important. In order to highlight the progress in clinical epilepsy research using modern methods of structural and functional imaging, some examples of this kind of advanced clinical research are given, such as prediction of postsurgical memory following temporal lobe surgery. Progress in the field of advanced EEG analysis is exemplified by EEG studies using non-linear analyses methods.

What do I expect for the future? Molecular biology and genetic research will further increase in basic experimental epilepsy research, and this will be paralleled by refinement of high tech imaging on the more clinical side. Furthermore, mechanisms of drug resistance to antiepileptic drugs can now be studied and this kind of research will increase.

As a consequence of better understanding the basic mechanisms of human epilepsy, new therapeutic treatment options, such as multiple subpial transection, vagus nerve stimulation, and high-frequency stimulation, have already emerged. Further studies are needed to elucidate their mechanisms and to establish firm and accepted indications. As a consequence of advanced medical technology, less invasive treatment, such as Gamma Knife treatment of epilepsies, has started to compete with classical neurosurgical interventions. Certainly more research in this area is necessary.

Basic Studies in the Context of Epilepsy Surgery and Presurgical Evaluation: Epileptogenesis and "Epileptic Circuits" in Mesial Temporal Lobe Epilepsy

Epilepsy surgery is "a window to the brain". It offers not only the unique opportunity to examine the basic mechanisms of epileptogenesis, but also allows the comparison of macroscopic and histologic structural changes to altered/disturbed EEG and behavioral function (anatomo-electro-clinical correlation). Today basic research in the laboratory is done on several levels: on the level of the single cell, as well as on the neuronal assembly and circuits. Since resected human tissue can be functionally examined over hours, it is now possible to study elementary processes of complex human performances.

Concerning basic research, the measurement of neurotransmitters and/or their precursors in chronic focal epilepsy was a milestone in modern epilepsy research. Studies of the last two decades, however, have shown that the absolute amounts of transmitters are less important. What turned out to be of utmost importance is the knowledge of the location of synapses, which are usually on aberrant dendritic sites. Modern research concentrates on the way how receptors and their subunit configurations are altered.

Pharmacotherapy refractory mesial temporal lobe epilepsy (MTLE) is the most common and therefore best studied epilepsy in epilepsy surgery series. It is associated with hippocampal sclerosis (HS). In the epileptic human hippocampus, there is neuronal loss and reactive gliosis in all fields of Ammon's horn and fascia dentata. The greatest cell losses are in areas CA1 (Sommer's sector) and prosubiculum. Usually the anterior hippocampus is more severely affected than the posterior part. In the synaptically reorganized fascia dentata and hippocampus, the mossy fiber sprout and hyperinnervate dendrites previously denervated as a consequence of cell losses that occur in HS.

Mossy fibers arise from granule cells and secrete glutamate aberrantly. They provide both monosynaptic *feedback* excitation on the dendrites of the granular cells and monosynaptic *feedforward* excitation on the hippocampal pyramidal cell dendrites. These abnormal circuits provide both increased number of glutamate axons and increased densities of the "rapid opening" AMPA (alpha-aminoisoxazole propionic acid)-sensitive-glutamate receptors. All this leads to enhanced amounts and enhanced synchrony of glutamate circuits which leads to enhanced temporal and spatial summation, mechanisms that are important for seizure generation. The glutamate receptor subtype NMDA (N-methyl-d-aspartate) is increased in granule cell reorganized epileptic circuits, further enhancing postsynaptic excitatory duration. NMDA receptor "dependent" prolonged burst firing has been demonstrated in in vitro recordings from human epileptic granule cells with mossy fibers synaptic reorganization [4].

Concerning inhibition the situation was less clear: Some authors argued that inhibition might be more or less intact in TLE, others argued that inhibitory mechanisms are important, because they contribute to the synchrony needed in cell-sparse hippocampal sclerosis [4]. Relying on recent literature for human tissue and animal models of TLE, it seems fairly established that there is impaired inhibitory neurotransmission in TLE. Evidence from human studies suggests that postsynaptic $GABA_A$ receptors contribute to the pathophysiology of MTLE with HS.

Zurich Contributions

In 1986 we studied the distribution of glutamic acid decarboxylase (GAD) immunoreactive neurons, fibres and punctae in sector CA1 of the adult human Ammon's horn in vibratome sections of tissue obtained at surgery [10]. The antibody was visualized by the unlabelled antibody enzyme method. The findings showed that GAD-immunoreactive neurons, fibres and punctae were present in all layers, however, most immunoreactive neurons were located in the stratum pyramidale and stratum lacunosum. Their size ranged from 8 microns in the stratum lacunosum to about 50 microns in the stratum oriens. All GAD-immunoreactive somata belonged to the heterogeneous group of non-pyramidal neurons. Within the stratum pyramidale all somata belonged to the group of lipofuscin-laden non-pyramidal neurons. The highest density of GAD-immunoreactive punctae was found in the stratum lacunosum.

In 1994 in an *in situ* hybridization histochemistry study, we demonstrated that excitatory amino acid AMPA receptor mRNA localization is affected in several regions of the human brain in epilepsy. In fact, an increase of the mRNA coding for the four AMPA receptor subunits in the hippocampus of epileptics was observed. The changes were most prominent in the granule cells of the dentate gyrus and most prominent for AMPA-B subunits [33].

During invasive Stereo-EEG presurgical evaluation in candidates for epilepsy surgery, we examined extracellular fluid from the primary epileptogenic area with push-pull cannulas inserted into the lumen of special hollow-core multicontact depth electrodes [16]. One minute fractionated samples of extracellular fluid were sequentially collected at a flow rate of 20 ul/min over a period of 1 hour and analyzed by o-phtalaldehyde precolumn derivatization high performance liquid chromatography (HPLC). Aspartate, glutamate, homocysteate, glycine, GABA, Beta-alanine, and taurine were detected at the femtomole level, and their profiles were plotted. Computer-assisted analyses of the background depth EEG (using compressed spectral array) and of spontaneous and electrically provoked epileptiform events (using automatic spike detection algorithms) were performed. The results were compared with the biochemical measurements. For two (out of three) patients a modulation of the aspartate level (from about 40 pmol/min to 70 pmol/min) was observed that correlated with the epileptiform EEG events. Non-transmitter amino acids remained unaffected [108, 19, 21].

In an ongoing study we try to determine whether and how $GABA_A$ receptor subtypes are altered. Loup *et al.* [56, 57] analyzed subunit composition and distribution of the three major $GABA_A$ receptor subtypes immunohistochemically with subunit-specific antibodies (α1, α2, α3, β2,3, and γ2) in surgical specimens from TLE patients with hippocampal sclerosis. Profound alterations in $GABA_A$ receptor subtype expression were observed when compared with control hippocampi. A decreased $GABA_A$ receptor subunit staining, reflecting cell loss, was observed in CA1, CA3, and hilus. In surviving neurons, the distinct neuron-specific expression pattern of the α-subunit variants observed in controls was markedly changed. In granule cells, prominent upregulation mainly of the α2-subunit was seen on somata and apical dendrites with reduced labeling on basal dendrites. In CA2, differential rearrangement of all three α-subunits occurred. Moreover, there was layer-specific loss of α1-subunit-immunoreactive interneurons in hippocampus proper, whereas surviving interneurons exhibited extensive changes in dendritic morphology. Expression patterns of β2,3- and γ2-subunits largely followed those of α-subunit variants. These results demonstrated a unique subtype-specific expression of $GABA_A$ receptors in human hippocampus. Furthermore, the significant reorganization of distinct receptor subtypes in surviving hippocampal neurons of TLE patients with hippocampal sclerosis, underlines the potential for synaptic plasticity in the human GABA system.

Migrational Disorders

Cortical dysplasia was first described by Taylor and co-workers [95]. It is now defined as neuronal migration disorder and cerebral or synaptic dysgenesis. It is a structural abnormality of cerebral cortex characterized by neuronal dyslamination. In its most severe form cytological features of neuron cell body enlargement and "dysmorphism" are present. Often cytoskeletal aberrations as well as proliferation of gemistocyte-like "balloon cells" among the bizarre neuronal perikarya are found [37]. The neuropathological features of some forms of severe cortical dysplasia suggest a morphological link to CNS lesions ("tubers") encountered in the multisystem neurocutaneous tuberous sclerosis. Tuberous sclerosis is the neurocutaneous disorder with the most consistent association with severe epilepsy [99].

A recently proposed classification system of neuronal migration disorders is based on three key events in formation of the cortex; (i) cellular (neuronal precursor) proliferation in the germinal matrix, (ii) neuronal precursor migration to the developing neocortex, and (iii) vertical and horizontal organisation of cells within the cortex with establishment of axonal and dendritic ramifications [5]. Some authors have proposed to define cortical dysplasia with balloon cells as a distinct tuberous sclerosis-related lesion subset [11].

Cellular/molecular genetic studies in the pathogenesis of cortical dysplasia and cortical tubers (which are seizure-generating lesions), have been stipulated by the discovery of the genes implicated in tuberous sclerosis. TSC2, localized to chromosome 16p13.3, encodes a 5.5-kilobase transcript and a protein, *tuberin*, widely expressed within various cultured cell lines and human viscera and CNS (neurons, choroid plexus, and ependyma). The protein is overexpressed in dysmorphic neurons, cortical tubers, and foci of sporadic cortical dysplasia. TSC1, a gene on chromosome 9q34, encodes a widely expressed 8.6-kilobase transcript that is translated into *hamartin*. Studies of the role of tuberous sclerosis-related genes in normal/abnormal cerebral growth and maturation may serve as a paradigm for examining the neurobiology of other epilepsy-determining genes (e.g. LIS-1, associated with lissencephaly). A methodology allowing for detailed analysis of unique transcript combinations within single cells of dysplastic cortex and tubers is now available [17].

Abnormalities of neuro-glia interactions, Cajal-Retzius cells, and transduction of calcium signals during cell migration to the cortex may play a role in the evolution of cortical dysplasia [31]. Dysregulation of inhibitors of programmed cell death (bcl-2, bcl-xL) may contribute to hamartomatous proliferation of neuronal precursors in cortical dysplasia [114]. Radiation of pregnant rats or transplacental exposure to methylazoxymethanol are potentially useful animal models to study epileptogenesis in these cortical malformations [34, 86]. A recent study by Zhu and Roper [116] showed reduced inhibition in an animal model of cortical dysplasia.

Studies of cortical dysplasia resected in humans suffering from pharmacotherapy resistent epilepsy, have suggested that epileptogenicity of dysplastic regions may be associated with the presence of NMDAR2 subunits and selectively expressed NMDAR1 splice variants in dysplastic neurons [115]. Other relevant findings are prominent $GABA_A$ beta immunoreactivity in the cytoplasm of dysmorphic neurons, and increased immunoreactivity with antisera to GluR1 and GluR2/3 glutamate receptors [99]. Also, staining of dysmorphic neurons for NMDAR2 has been found [50]. Recent studies showed selective alterations in glutamate and GABA receptor subunit mRNA expression in dysplastic neurons and giant cells of cortical tubers [112, 18]. Less clear is the role of peptide neurotransmitters in cortical dysplasia. Nevertheless, some immunocytochemistry studies with neuropeptide Y, parvalbumin and calbindin-D28k have been undertaken [99].

Cortical malformations show signs of intrinsic epileptogenicity [72]. At present, the mechanisms of this epileptogenicity are still not adequately understood. Metabolic investigations of these malformations in vivo during interictal and ictal state with magnetic resonance spectroscopy (^{1}H-MRS) and PET may help to elucidate some of these mechanisms. Hammers *et al.* [43] studied the $GABA_A$ central benzodiazepine receptors in malformations of cortical development by PET ([^{11}C]flumazenil volume of distribution = [^{11}C]FMZ-Vd) and found in 9 out of 10 patients single or multiple increases of [^{11}C]FMZ-Vd. Using α[^{11}C]methyl-L-tryptophan PET, Chugani *et al.* [15] were able to image and differentiate epileptogenic tubers with tuberous sclerosis.

Migrational Disorders: What do I Expect for the Future?

(1) The development of animals in which both TSC1 and TSC2 homolog genes are mutated or deleted ("knockout").
(2) Engineering of neuronal precursors (e.g. NT2 cells) in tissue culture a) to overexpress tubarin/hamartin, b) to study effects on cell proliferation, migration, and differentiation; and c) for comparable studies with other broadly defined cortical-dysplasia – associated genes (e.g. LIS-1).
(3) Direct electrophysiological recordings from cortical dysplastic lesions during presurgical evaluation and from dysmorphic neuroglial cells in corticectomy specimen to clarify their contribution to seizure genesis.
(4) In vivo 1H-MRS and PET studies of patients with migrational disorders, combined with histological and immunohistological studies to correlate the findings, and to elucidate some of these epileptogenic mechanisms.

Zurich Contributions

Interictal and Ictal MRS in Cortical Dysgenesis. Recently we reported the magnetic resonance imaging (MRI) and proton magnetic resonance spectroscopic findings (^{1}H-MRS) in a patient with a focal cortical dysgenesis, in the right superior frontal gyrus during intermittent frontal status epilepticus (IFSE) with simple partial seizures, and after she had become seizure free [61].

During the status epilepticus, demonstrated by simultaneous behavioural and electroencephalographic telemetric long-term monitoring with scalp electrodes and ictal SPECT, we performed a single voxel spectroscopy of the dysgenic cortex. The ^{1}H-MRS was repeated after 20 days when the patient's seizures were controlled. We found that the N-acetyl-aspartate (NAA) concentration in the focal dysgenic cortex was decreased in the interictal state, but more during IFSE. The creatine/phosphocreatine (Cr) concentration was normal in both instances. There was a clear lactate signal during IFSE, which was no longer visible in the interictal state. The observed changes were interpreted as signs of histopathological changes inherent to a cortical malformation and of an impaired energy metabolism due to the partial status epilepticus.

NAA is conventionally considered to be a marker of functional neurons in the adult brain. A reduction of NAA is usually interpreted as reduced neuronal density and/or neuronal dysfunction. We showed that the reduction of the NAA-signal in the region of the focal cortical dysgenesis was more marked during the IFSE. Thus, NAA reductions after a seizure do not necessarily reflect an irreversible neuronal loss, but can also be a marker of a reversible neuronal dysfunction.

The theory of an impaired energy metabolism during IFSE is supported by the lactate-signal in the ictal spectra, which was no longer visible in the interictal spectra. An ictal and post-ictal increase of lactate, not only in the epileptogenic focus but also in the projection areas, was also observed in animal studies dependent on the duration and severity of seizures [77, 65, 66, 58]. It has been assumed that the lactate accumulation after seizures reflects a mismatch between glycolysis and oxidative metabolism, or a temporary dysequilibrium between lactate production and clearance [1, 78]. Interestingly, the lactate increase could not be demonstrated consistently in ictal studies in humans. The enhanced visibility of choline indicating an accumulation of phospholipid breakdown products may be viewed as an argument for an impaired energy metabolism; this is because phospholipid synthesis is an energy demanding process depending on mitochondrial metabolism.

Proton Magnetic Resonance Spectroscopy

Zurich Contributions

Hippocampal Sclerosis (HS) in MTLE. In a pilot study we determined the value of in vivo ^{1}H-MRS for diagnosing HS in MTLE. We measured hippocampal metabolite concentrations by localized in vivo ^{1}H-MRS in 11 patients suffering from refractory MTLE, as well as in 11 age-matched healthy volunteers. These metabolites were compared with patient history, postoperative outcome and histopathology [25]. Main results of this study were that in patients, the decrease in NAA concentrations was highly significant ipsilateral, and less but still significant contralateral to the electroencephalographically defined primary epileptogenic area, as compared to controls. Furthermore, the decrease in ipsilateral NAA measured preoperatively correlated well with the degree of HS, but did not reliably predict postoperative outcome. Nevertheless there was a trend toward better outcome in patients with a marked decrease of NAA. In this study hippocampal NAA decrease (ipsi- and contralateral) was highly correlated with early onset age of epileptic seizures. We found a strong association between duration of the disease and contralateral (and, though less clear-cut, ipsilateral) NAA loss. These results supported the notion of a generally progressive course of poorly controlled MTLE.

Brain Glutathione Levels in Epilepsy. Recently Müller *et al.* [62] studied brain glutathione levels in patients with epilepsy measured by in vivo ^{1}H-MRS technique developed in Zurich. Measurements of glutathione levels were performed in structurally normal-appearing tissue in the parietooccipital region of each hemisphere in patients with and without active epilepsy, and in an age-matched control group. (Volume of interest $25 \times 25 \times 25$ mm). Compared to healthy controls, in epileptic patients the GSH/water ratio was significantly reduced in both hemispheres, i.e. we found evidence for a widespread impairment of the glutathione system in epileptic patients. This is of interest because (a) glutathione in its reduced form (GSH) is the most important free radical scavenging compound in the mammalian nervous system that prevents membrane lipid peroxidation, and (b) it is suspected that epileptic seizures are accompanied by a massive production of reactive oxygen species, i.e. oxidative stress.

Prediction of Responders to Treatment with GABA-Ergic Antiepileptic Drugs. Mueller *et al.* [63] studied the effects of vigabatrin (VGB) by measuring the GABA (γ-aminobutyric acid) and homocarnosine/creatine and phosphocreatine ratio (GABA+/Cr) (+ denotes the contamination with macromolecules) by means of ^{1}H-MRS. The purpose of the study was to identify possible responders before or in an early phase of VGB treatment. Measurements were performed in 14 patients with drug-resistant TLE and 3 patients with occipital lobe epilepsy. GABA+/Cr was measured in the ipsilateral (i.e. epileptogenic) hemisphere and contralateral (i.e. nonepileptogenic) hemisphere in a volume of 8 cm^3. VGB increases the human brain (GABA) level by irreversibly inhibiting GABA transaminase. Although some patients respond to VGB with a significant seizure reduction others do not. In this study, measurements were taken immediately before and after a titration period of 1 month (VGB 2 g/day during the past 2 weeks). A third measurement followed after a maintenance period of 3 months (VGB 2 or 3 g/day). Depending on the therapeutic efficacy of VGB, three groups were defined: (a) full responders, (b) nonresponders, and (c) partial responders. The nonresponders showed no significant change in the GABA+/Cr signal during the treatment compared with baseline. The full responders had a significant increase of the GABA+/Cr signal during the whole treatment phase and a lower ipsilateral level at baseline. The partial responders also had a lowered ipsilateral GABA+/Cr signal at baseline and an increase during treatment but a decrease when the seizures started again. We concluded that responders to

VGB treatment could be identified by a lower ipsilateral baseline GABA+/Cr signal and a steeper increase during VGB treatment.

In a related MRS study we examined the *influence of pyridoxal 5′-phosphate (PP) alone and in combination with various doses of VGB on brain GABA levels* [64]. Both iso-forms of the GABA synthesising enzyme and also the GABA degrading enzyme need PP as coenzyme. The aim was to investigate the influence of PP alone and in combination with various doses of VGB on brain GABA levels. In 8 healthy subjects, 300 mg/d PP and various doses of VGB (range 1000 mg/d to 4000 mg/d) were given alone or in combination. The GABA+/creatine (Cr) signals in both occipital lobes were measured before treatment, during monotherapy with PP or VGB, and during combination of both using ^{1}H-MRS. PP alone did not change the GABA+/Cr signals. VGB alone increased the GABA+/Cr signals in both hemispheres. The combination PP and low-medium dosed VGB (1000–2000 mg/d) did not increase the GABA+/Cr signals. The effects of the combination of PP and high dosed (3000–4000 mg/d) VGB on the GABA+/Cr signals varied depending on the sequence of the drugs and the dose of VGB. We concluded that the combination of PP and low-high dosed VGB had inconsistent effects on the GABA+/Cr signals compared to a VGB monotherapy because PP activates also the GABA-degrading enzyme GABA-transaminase. This finding is also of interest regarding etiology and treatment of pyridoxal-phosphate dependent seizures.

Rasmussen's Encephalitis

Rasmussen's encephalitis (RE) is a rare but devastating form of childhood epilepsy. It is characterized by progressive, inflammatory destruction of a single cerebral hemisphere, associated with intractable focal seizures and loss of function in the affected hemisphere. In the early phase of the disease, histopathological observations include a pronounced perivascular inflammation, reactive microglia, and neuronophagia. In the chronic phase of the disease, symptoms include microglial nodules, little inflammation, and tissue destruction with gliosis in the affected hemisphere [79, 84, 49, 30]. Functional hemispherectomy is the recommended therapy [80, 69]. In a subgroup of patients, treatment with corticosteroids and intravenous immunoglobulin has ameliorated the state of disease [100, 44].

In recent years it has been suggested that RE could be an autoimmune disease because circulating factors, likely autoantibodies to glutamate receptor subunit GluR3, are pathogenic in at least some patients with RE. The presence of antibodies to the glutamate receptor subunit GluR3 in RE patients prompted therapeutic trials with plasmapheresis, and transient beneficial therapeutic effects have been observed [85, 2, 97].

The autoimmune concept of RE derived from experiments in which rabbits were immunized with a portion of the rat AMPA-type glutamate receptor subunit GluR3 (amino acids 245–457). They developed typical seizures and histopathologic features mimicking Rasmussen's encephalitis. Moreover, antibodies against rat GluR3 were found by immunoblot analysis and immunocytochemistry on transfected HEK 293 cells in two patient sera, and a correlation was noticed between serum titers of GluR3 antibodies and frequency of seizures in one of these patients [85]. Furthermore, rabbit anti-GluR$3_{245–457}$ antisera and RE patient serum elicited currents in cultured mouse cortical neurons that could be blocked by a competitive AMPA receptor antagonist. These antisera and IgG evoked currents could be specifically blocked by a synthetic peptide prepared to subregion GluR3B (amino acids 372–395) [97]. In another study, rabbits immunized with a fusion protein containing GluR$3_{246–455}$ developed a neurological disorder similar to Rasmussen's encephalitis. Their sera triggered neuronal cell death in rat cortical cultures by a complement-dependent mechanism but did not evoke glutamate receptor activity in such neurons [45].

On the other hand, RE cases with no detectable anti-GluR antibodies were described, including a patient (29 years old) who was highly responsive to immunosuppressive treatment [3, 51]. Hence, the cause of RE is still uncertain. This raises the following questions: Does an autoantibody mechanism cause RE? and: Does the RE-like symptomatic rabbit represent an appropriate experimental model of the disease manifested in RE patients [70]?

Zurich Contributions

Together with the research group of Streit [96] we have studied histologically verified RE patients and some patients with suspected immune-mediated epilepsies. In various assay systems, we tested for the presence of anti-GluR3 autoantibodies in sera and CSF of the RE patients and controls. We used immunocyto-chemistry on HEK 293 and COS-7 cells that expressed GluR3 following transient transfection. Immunoreactivity was also assessed by immunoblotting experiments on extracts from such cells and from rat or calf brain. This was performed by a histoblotting procedure on material from rat brain sections and by a dot assay on synthetic peptides that represent the sequence domain GluR3. Until now, with CSF, sera and immunoglobulin preparations from the 3 RE patients we examined, no specific signals or patterns of immunoreactivity could be detected in any of the assay systems. However, a monoclonal antibody recognizing GluR2/3, which was used for control, yielded robust signals in the immunocytochemical and immunoblotting assays. These results suggest that there are several forms of Rasmussen's encephalitis, with and without autoantibodies to GluR3.

One of the most interesting findings of this otherwise negative study was derived from the histoblot procedure in which material from rat brain sections was transferred onto nitrocellulose membranes and immunostained. Streit's group applied this technique to determine whether potential staining patterns corresponded to the distribution of GluR3 protein, since knowledge about the distribution of GluR3 in rat brain had been established at the transcript level. Streit and co-workers found that the histoblot labeling pattern obtained with the monoclonal anti-GluR2/3 antibody, mAb 1F1, seemed to correspond well to the sum of the distribution patterns of GluR2 and GluR3 proteins. Whilst with the sera of the 3 RE patients no distinctive labeling patterns were generated, the serum of a control patient (MB), who did not suffer from RE but rather from an unclassifiable form of epilepsy, produced a striking staining pattern in histoblots. In the hippocampal formation, this pattern was reminiscent of immunocytochemical staining patterns for glutamate or of uptake patterns for D-aspartate, a false transmitter that is transported by the same high-affinity uptake system as L-glutamate [94, 38]. Thus, we had to conclude that antibodies in the serum of patient MB recognized a rat brain protein. In fact, this serum also produced a histoblot staining pattern in human cerebellar cortex that was characterized by strong labeling of the molecular layer as seen in the rat cerebellum (B. Stierli and P. Streit, unpublished observations).

The relationship between these serum antibodies and the disease of patient MB remains unknown. At present, these interesting findings have research implications for putative immune-mediated epilepsies.

Functional Outcome Prediction

Risk Factors Associated with Postsurgical Decrements in Memory

Decrements in memory function continue to be a frequent complication of temporal lobe (TL) surgery. Side of surgery, extent of resection, structural and functional adequacy, age of seizure onset, age at time of surgery and gender differences have all been identified as potential risk factors [14]. Therefore, prediction of memory outcome following TL surgery is of paramount importance.

Zurich Contributions

Epilepsy surgery involving functionally important areas requires careful presurgical functional studies. With respect to the role of the hippocampal formation in learning and memory we have undertaken several clinical studies *comparing pre- and postoperative learning and memory performances* after selective amygdalohippocampectomy (AHE) [107]. We tried to correlate the results with the preoperative state, the underlying pathology, and the extent of resection. These studies can be summarized as follows: (1) In patients with a marked pre-operative unilateral material-specific deficit, no or only a minor postoperative decline of memory function for material specific for the operated hemisphere was found; (2) the neuropsychological deficits of these patients were more marked after left compared to right AHE; (3) in general, there was a strong positive correlation between (a) postoperative memory performance and seizure outcome and, (b) severity of neuropathological findings (neuronal loss, degree of hippocampal sclerosis, and severity of microdysgenesis). A strong correlation was also found between postoperative seizure outcome and postoperative neuropsychological outcome; (4) the extent of resection, in particular the extent of the removal of the parahippocampal gyrus, is also an important variable in terms of postsurgical memory outcome; (5) long-term neuropsychological follow-up data are better for the AHE group compared to that of an earlier series with classical anterior 2/3 temporal lobe resection [9].

For patients at risk we have developed selective amobarbital tests. The classical intracarotid Wada-test allows for speech lateralisation and to a certain degree for prediction of memory performance following unilateral TL resection. An exact prediction of the postoperative memory performance following a unilateral AHE turned out to be very difficult using the intracarotid Wada-test. Since 1986, we have developed and steadily improved the so-called *selective temporal lobe amobarbital memory tests* (STLAMT) [109]. Initially three methods were used: (1) the so-called temporary balloon occlusion distal to the origin of the anterior choroidal artery, with injection of Amobarbital into the anterior choroidal artery and the posterior communicating artery (as well as into the ophthalmic artery), (2) the superselective injection of Amobarbital into the anterior choroidal artery, and (3) the injection of amobarbital into the P2 segment of the posterior cerebral artery. With behavioral and EEG-monitoring (preferentially with foramen ovale- and/or depth electrodes), the co-injection of amobarbital and SPECT-tracer (HMPAO) and subsequent SPECT allow for a precise determination of the inactivated structures.

Up to now 89 *selective Amobarbital tests* have been performed at the University Zürich. With a few exceptions of selective inactivations of language areas [39] these were STLAMT. In the majority, the selective catheterization of the anterior choroidal artery was preferred. We had no complications. STLAMT allows for a reliable prediction of postoperative memory performance following selective amygdalohippocampectomy (AHE). The described refinements enable us to interpret individual test data with high confidence.

The best way to predict possible deficits associated with the resection is temporary inactivation of the structures intended to be definitively resected. The selective inactivation of the territory of the anterior choroidal artery is very useful to predict memory outcome in candidates for AHE [104]. Nevertheless the variability of the vascular supply of the hippocampal formation may present problems. Therefore, the appropriate interpretation of the task-performance asks for co-injection of a SPECT tracer and concomitant EEG-recording from the structures of interest.

With (used in Zürich) dual verbal and non-verbal coding recurrent memory task the prediction of postoperative memory performance (using nonverbal motor responses, i.e. button press) is rather good for the verbal memory. On the other hand, it underestimates postoperative non-verbal (figural) memory performance [109].

Event-Related Potential Studies on the Role of Mesial Temporal Lobe Structures in Memory

The advantages of EEG and event-related potentials (ERPs) are their great temporal resolution and direct relation to neuronal-information processing. Successive ERP components are related to successive stages in information processing, from a strictly sensory to the highest integrative levels, termed "endogenous". If the intracranial generators of scalp ERP components can be identified, then the intensity, onset and duration of activation of specific brain systems involved in a task can be non-invasively monitored. The process of estimating cerebral generators from observed scalp ERP topography is "solving the inverse problem". Cognitive Event-Related Potentials (CERPs) are generated by extended surfaces in multiple brain areas, rather than by a simple dipole, therefore intracerebral recordings yield the best information. Within the intracerebrally recorded CERPs, four main areas are of interest; (1) potentials to rare target and distractor auditory and visual stimuli; (2) modality-specific responses to rarity, including the so-called P3a and P3b systems; (3) CERPs to novel and repeated words and figures, and; (4) other late CERPs, such as the CNV, and the RP (Bereitschafts-Potential, "readiness-potential").

Of particular interest for orientation of attention are the P3a system and the P3b event-encoding system. The P3a system is mainly located in the inferior parietal, cingulate, and dorsolateral prefrontal cortex; the P3b system in the hippocampus, superior temporal sulcus, lateral orbito-frontal cortex, and intraparietal sulcus [41, 42].

In TLE patients, intracranial CERPs show alterations (increase in latency and decrease of amplitude), which correlate well with the Wechsler Memory Scale, and the hippocampal P300 correlates well with neuronal cell density. The recently described N400 recorded from the anterior fusiform gyrus is thought to reflect access of semantic memory, whereas the P300 is thought to reflect rules-based mapping of stimuli onto discrete covert or overt responses, i.e. encoding processes [67, 59, 68]. Paller *et al.* [71] found that late potentials around 500–900 ms account for the subject's engagement in recollection processing. ERPs differentiate priming and recognition to familiar and unfamiliar faces [7]. Several authors described limbic correlates of the scalp P300 elicited in visual and auditory odd-ball paradigms using depth electrodes in epileptic patients [40, 41, 42, 89, 55, 36] and to the scalp N400 in word recognition paradigms [36]. Therefore it can be assumed that the careful study of ERPs recorded from mesiobasal temporal structures in TLE patients has the potential to clarify the role of these structures in the various kinds of memory and to quantify preoperative deficits. Indeed, Grunwald *et al.* [36] recently reported that the amplitude of the intrahippocampal N400 elicited in a word recognition paradigm is an excellent predictor of postoperative memory performance in patients suffering from temporal lobe epilepsy.

Zurich Contributions. Recently, Stephan Wieser completed an ERP study [111] in which Henke's paradigm [46, 47, 48] was used, examining episodic memory with the associative word learning task (AWL); the semantic memory with the deep single word encoding task (DSWE) and the explicit memory with the shallow single word encoding task (SSWE). ERP correlates of encoding and retrieval and behavioral data were analysed. EEG was taken conventionally (10/20 system). Scalp electrodes were placed in healthy subjects. Foramen ovale electrodes were placed in patients with MTLE who underwent presurgical evaluation.

A crucial question of this study was whether an electrophysiological correlate of building associations could be found. The ERPs in the task condition with associative binding (AWL) and without (DSWE) were compared. We found such an effect reflected by a positivity in the time window 400–600 ms with a significant predominance over the left hemisphere. This result supports the "association-hypothesis" [47] without giving the close link to hippocampal formation, suggesting a more widely distributed memory system with some kind of lateralization to the left hemisphere.

Concerning *retrieval*, the recollection of associatively learned word pairs generated significantly different ERP components from 200–1000 ms compared to the other word learning conditions i.e. both shallow and deep single word encoding (SSWE and DSWE). This evidence for different memory mechanisms fits well with previous work. Another most intriguing finding with regard to retrieval was that there was no difference between ERPs elicited by retrieval of the word pairs, learned by single item encoding using language processing strategies (DSWE), compared to that without (SSWE). This result was unexpected. That is, these word pairs were not only learned by different strategies but also have different underlying encoding processes. These processes are clearly reflected in the different ERP components during encoding. This finding suggests that once stored, both kinds of information are recollected in the same way. Access to stored information is independent of learning strategies excepting associative binding. In PET studies, associative binding has been attributed to the hippocampal formation [46].

The hippocampal formation has been identified as a crucial structure for the P3b event encoding system [41, 42]. Therefore, we studied epileptic patients who had foramen ovale (FO) electrodes allowing us to record directly from the mesiotemporal lobe. Most interestingly, in the FO electrode recorded patient data, there was a clear-cut gradient for ERP *encoding* components. The largest test effects were found in the anterior FO electrode contacts of the "healthy" side. These results are in concordance with the so-called HIPER model. This model is derived from a meta-analysis of PET-studies that demonstrate that the the encoding system is assigned to the anterior hippocampal formation [53].

In line with ERP and fMRI *"Remember-Know"* studies we found that correctly recognized old word pairs (hits) recalled with autonoetic awareness ("remember") generate different ERPs than those remembered with noetic awareness ("know"). Differing electrophysiological correlates were identified for the two states of consciousness. This study has provided evidence that different components of memory, i.e. encoding and retrieval mechanisms, are reflected in behavioral and task-specific ERP correlates. In contrast to fMRI and PET studies, this electrophysiological study provides additional insight in the dynamic aspects of the various, previously hypothesized memory subsystems, including associative, semantic and implicit memory.

Zurich $H_2{}^{15}O$ *PET Studies for Memory Assessment.* Several PET experiments were aimed at defining the role(s) of the hippocampal formations in memory [46, 47, 48]. Mesial temporal lobe epilepsy (MTLE) patients have been examined before and 6–9 months after AHE with $H_2{}^{15}O$ PET. In addition concurrent EEG registration was documented while they were performing hippocampus sensitive memory tasks. The preoperative PET and EEG examinations during memory tasks included the recording from bilaterally implanted foramen ovale electrodes. These electrodes were situated below each hippocampal formation. PET analysis was performed with 3 scans per condition per patient. Group analyses included the within-subject comparison pre- to postoperative in patients with either a right or left side AHE.

The PET analyses have demonstrated that our PET protocol is sensitive enough to spot hippocampal blood flow changes in individual patients; in addition, they show that the postoperative reorganization of hippocampus-dependent memory functions can involve the compensatory effort of the contralateral (healthy) hippocampus in patients with no memory loss. This is in line with the observation that in several patients who underwent AHE on the left side the verbal memory and intelligence were unchanged pre- to postoperatively while the nonverbal memory improved considerably.

Zurich $H_2{}^{15}O$ *PET Studies for Assessment of Motor Functions.* Reorganization of motor functions were studied in several patients with Rasmussen's encephalitis, particularly in a woman with Rasmussen's encephalitis after limited Rolandic resection before the necessary hemispherectomy with $H_2{}^{15}O$ PET. These studies showed that the ipsilateral corticospinal tract of the healthy hemisphere had compensated for the lost contralateral motor innervation [110].

Zurich Functional MR (fMRI) and Intraoperative Cortical Stimulation Studies in Patients with Lesions in or Close to the Rolandic Cortex

Fandino *et al.* [29] compared the results of fMRI with those of intraoperative electrocorticography (ECoG) and direct electrical cortical stimulation (ECS) in patients with tumors in or near the Rolandic cortex. Patients had presurgically blood oxygen level-dependent (BOLD) fMRI using a T2-weighted, echo planar acquisition on a 1.5-T MR imager, while performing a motor paradigm consisting of clenching and spreading of the hand contra- and ipsilateral to the tumor. Statistical cross-correlation functional maps covering the primary and secondary motor cortex (resolution 3,1 × 3,1 × 5 mm) were generated and overlaid onto MR images.

Patients were operated under general anesthesia using short-acting relaxants, propofol and no barbiturates. Intraoperative ECoG and cortical stimulation (Ojemann Cortical Stimulator; bipolar square-wave pulses of 1 to 4 ms, 50 and 60 Hz, beginning with a current of 2 mA [up to 10 mA, if necessary]) with a bipolar probe and using strip electrodes was performed in all patients. Topographical mapping of spikes and slow delta waves was done. Stimulation sites were topographically analyzed with respect to positive motor responses and after discharges.

fMRI showed signal intensity changes in the range of 2% to 5% between rest and activation conditions in all patients. In 6/8 patients the anatomical fMRI localization was verified by the results of ECS. In 2/8 patients motor responses were obtained from other regions than that predicted by fMRI, and ECS of the fMRI determined region was negative. We conclude that fMRI provides useful information for surgery in motor brain areas. In our small series the correlation between fMRI and results of ECS was significant although not 100%.

Seizure Prediction

The domain of EEG with all its related fields is an integral part of most clinical and research laboratories. Albeit in hot competition with fMRI, PET and MRS, its computerized quantification with all sophisticated modern ramifications promise that the EEG will be playing a major role in the future. This is thanks to its most obvious advantages, the great *temporal resolution* and the *direct relation* to neuronal-information processing.

Epileptology is one of the areas, in which EEG is of paramount importance. Already the interictal EEG may show characteristic epileptiform transients, which in many instances allow for a classification of the type of epilepsy. Moreover, seizures usually express themselves in rather characteristic discharges in the EEG. With exception of the so-called reflex epilepsies, the occurrence of the seizures is considered to be at random and to a great deal unpredictable. Great hope is therefore laid in the possibility to forecast the occurrence of seizures from the EEG. Studies in this direction have already a long history, but were not very successful. Recently, however, the first reports were published showing that non-linear analysis methods of EEG might be more promising.

From a clinical point of view there exist several arguments which support the notion that at least certain seizures can be predicted. These are the existence of seizure facilitating factors on the one hand and seizure preventing strategies on the other as well as the existence of behavioral and/or autonomous nervous system prodromal changes in certain patients. Last but not least, the existence of prolonged aura states, i.e. the so-called *aura continua*, which is often terminated by an overt seizure, is ample evidence that the prediction of an impending seizure might be possible. "Support

Dogs", a registered charity, which trains dogs to assist disabled people, has successfully trained several "seizure-alert dogs". It was claimed that these dogs were able to warn accurately within time periods varying from 15 to 45 minutes, although this has never been explored scientifically [92].

Computational techniques of wave analysis started with the Fourier analysis, applied as early as 1932 by physicist Dietsch [20], a collaborator of Berger, culminating in the signal analysis using nonlinear methods of the so-called chaos theory. Condensed spectral array (CSA), phase- and coherence analysis [35], spectral edge frequency analysis [101] and some more advanced non-linear analysis methods [87, 54] have been used to study the transition of interictal to ictal state. Sherwin [88] and Lange *et al.* [52] showed that stronger coupling of certain hodologically related brain regions occur during a seizure which is paralleled by a decrease in degrees of freedom. Other studies have concentrated on changes of the shape of epileptiform potentials or evoked potentials with paroxysmal appearance (réponses paroxystiques, [12, 13]) during the course of a seizure, or during various different degrees of vigilance [103]. These changes may reflect different activity levels of spike producing neuronal populations and different states of connectivity of preferential pathways. Although preferential pathways basically reflect the anatomical hodology of the brain, they undergo dynamic kindling-like changes in the presence of an active epileptic process [13]. Studies on the recovery cycle with paired pulse stimulation brought some evidence that the autochthonous regional EEG rhythm bears some relations to the recovery cycle of a certain neuronal loop [103], and thus it may be reasonable to assume that the "excitability" state of a brain system is reflected in the subtle changes of the EEG rhythms.

In recent years microdialysis and push-pull cannula-device data have been linked with EEG analysis techniques and provided some insights into the neurochemical correlates of EEG changes preceding a seizure. The Yale group has presented interesting data obtained by human in vivo microdialysis of hippocampi during spontaneous seizures. Using this technique in epileptic patients who had depth electrodes implanted and were evaluated for epilepsy surgery, a basal glutamate increase of about 10% and a basal gamma-aminobutyric acid (GABA) decrease of about 25% were found in the epileptic hippocampus. *Prior to a seizure*, the glutamate rose in the epileptic hippocampus up to 100 μmol, a level at which neurotoxicity might occur. Furthermore the GABA rose higher contra-lateral to the epileptogenic hippocampus. These findings were interpreted as pointing to a GABA transporter problem [26].

Zurich Contributions

With regard to the attenuation (i.e. "flattening") phenomenon of background activity before seizures, we found that anodal polarization of limbic structures may lead to similar attenuation phenomena [105] raising the question of more general fundamental basic relationships between DC shifts, seizure facilitation/prevention and clinical correlates [91].

We studied the *effects of weak direct polarizing currents applied to the primary epileptogenic focus* before surgical removal of the amygdala and the hippocampal formation in three patients suffering from drug-resistant MTLE. The primary epileptogenic area responsible for the patient's habitual seizures had been previously localized with stereoelectroencephalography (SEEG). At the end of the SEEG-examination, when the depth electrodes were still *in situ*, weak DC currents were applied between poles situated either in the epileptogenic amygdala or the hippocampus and a large (5 × 5 cm) scalp electrode placed over the ipsilateral fronto-temporal scalp using a 9 V battery-powered constant-current device. This device allowed for continuous monitoring of current flow by an amperometer in series. The influence of the DC field on the spontaneously occurring EEG activity with focal epileptic spikes and the changes of evoked EEG responses recorded within the hippocampus and evoked by electrical 1/s pulse stimulation of the ipsilateral amygdala were studied. At each session we started with a low initial current flow of 1 μA for 10 seconds and carefully observed the EEG and the behavior of the patient.

Results of these experiments [90] can be summarized as follows: Anodal (positive pole) polarization decreased the epileptic spike incidence, while cathodal (negative pole) polarization had an opposite effect. Evoked potentials recorded from the hippocampus and elicited by electrical pulse stimulation of the ipsilateral amygdala were altered in shape by a weak, polarizing current and these effects were related to current intensity. Two patients were unable to tell whether they were under the influence of DC currents, however, in one patient a marked temporary behavioral alteration was observed following the polarization experiment, in the sense of an acute psychotic state [105].

The results of our more recent studies on the effects of weak DC electromagnetic fields on the EEG point to the same direction. Ten patients with MTLE were submitted to a standardized DC electromagnetic stimulation protocol with 1–3 mTesla field strength. A significant change in the rate of spikes (P value = 0.04) was noted in the case of stimulating for 30 seconds, with the gradient (as opposed to homogeneous) field configuration at a field strength of 3 mTesla. These pooled results were compared with individual data where the spikes were assessed by visual counting. It became obvious that only in 5 out of a total of 10 patients large differences in the spike frequency before and after stimulation were present, i.e. only half of the patients showed a clear-cut "electro-magnetic sensitivity". The results of this study are in agreement with the results reported in earlier studies [24, 32]. Further evidence, however, is needed to confirm the hypothesis that the intraparenchymatously found magnetizable particle (presumably magnetite and maghemite) concentration accounts for these phenomena [22, 23].

Lyapunov Spectra and Related Measures of Complexity in the EEG. Analysis methods of the EEG derived from the theory of nonlinear dynamics are able to give new insights into the dynamics of the EEG. Chaos indicators (Lyapunov exponents, correlation dimensions and related measures of complexity in the EEG) exhibit characteristic changes as a function of certain physiological and pathological brain states. Correlation dimension D2 and largest Lyapunov exponents decrease at onset and during seizures [28]. Seizure prediction, by calculating Lyapunov spectra, was possible in several off-line analyzed seizures. Interpretable alterations of the correlation dimension D2 appeared up to several minutes before clinical seizure onset [106].

In a replication study we investigated whether a correct lateralization of the primary epileptogenic area by means of neuronal complexity loss analysis can be obtained from interictal EEG recordings. Semi-invasive foramen ovale electrodes were used in this study [102]. The Bonn group used recordings from intrahippocampal depth and subdural strip electrodes to show that the dynamics of the primary epileptogenic area can be characterized by an increased loss of neuronal complexity, in patients with unilateral TLE. Neuronal complexity loss analysis was applied, derived from the theory of nonlinear dynamics.

Examining the interictal EEG recorded intracranially from multipolar foramen ovale electrodes in 19 patients with unilateral TLE undergoing presurgical evaluation, we found that the primary epileptogenic area was correctly lateralized in 16 of the 19 investigated patients.

New Therapeutic Options in Epilepsy Surgery

Besides multiple subpial transections (MST) [93], vagal nerve stimulation (VNS) [60, 113] high-frequency stimulation of the subthalamic nucleus [8] and of thalamic nuclei, as well as chronic electrical stimulation of the hippocampal formation [98] have been proposed.

Gamma Knife treatment of epilepsy has started to compete with open classical neurosurgical treatment options [81, 82, 83]. It is particularly in this area of research where the Graz group made pioneering contributions in the last years [73, 74, 75, 76, 6, 27].

Concluding Remarks

The primary goal of a causal (=curative) therapy of the epilepsies is the correction of the causes of the epilepsy syndrome. Unfortunately, at present, this is only possible to a limited extent. Much expectation lies in a) the discovery of the possible causes of resistance to common antiepileptic drugs (increased activity of P-glycoprotein drug efflux-pump in the epileptogenic focus); and b) the discovery of the pathophysiology of some epilepsy syndromes as autoimmune diseases, as well as in c) the better understanding of certain epilepsy syndromes as genetically determined aberrations. The biochemical in vivo characterization of certain epilepsy syndromes, has now become feasible by methods such as the noninvasive proton magnetic resonance spectroscopy. Technical advances, which might gain importance for epilepsy therapy in the near future, are 'radiosurgery' and probably also gene-therapy, i.e. the treatment of focal epilepsies by intracerebral grafting of GABA- and adenosine-releasing cells, developed in transgenic mice.

Acknowledgment

I am indebted to Mrs. Hariklia Proios, Research Scientist ETH Zurich, who improved the English; and to Mrs. Simone Spring, who helped with the references. I also wish to thank Drs. Fabienne Loup, Susanne Mueller, Stephan Wieser, Profs. Peter Streit and Jean-Marc Fritschy for helpful comments.

References

1. Ackermann RF, Lear JL (1989) Glycolysis-induced discordance between glucose metabolic rates measured with radiolabelled fluorodeoxyglucose and glucose. J Cereb Blood Flow Metab 6: 774–785
2. Andrews PI, Dichter MA, Berkovic SF, Newton MR, McNamara JO (1996) Plasmapheresis in Rasmussen's encephalitis. Neurology 46: 242–246
3. Antel JP, Rasmussen T (1996) Rasmussen's encephalitis and the new hat. Neurology 46: 9–11
4. Babb TL (2001) Research on neurotransmitters in human epileptic hippocampus. In: Lüders HO, Comair YG (eds) Epilepsy surgery, 2nd edn. Lippincott-Raven, Philadelphia, pp 935–940
5. Barkovich AJ, Kuzniecky RI, Dobyns WB, Jackson GD, Becker LE, Evrard P (1996) A classification scheme for malformations of cortical development. Neuropediatrics 27: 59–63
6. Bartolomei F, Régis J, Kida Y, Kobayashi T, Vladyka V, Liscak R, Forster D, Kemeny A, Schröttner O, Pendl G (1999) Gamma Knife radiosurgery for epilepsy associated with cavernous hemangiomas: a retrospective study of 49 cases. Stereotact Funct Neurosurg 72 [Suppl] 1: 22–28
7. Begleiter H, Porjesz B, Wang W (1995) Event-related brain potentials differentiate priming and recognition to familiar and unfamiliar faces. Electroencephalogr Clin Neurophysiol 94: 41–49
8. Benabid AL, Bressand K, Vercueil L, Dematteis M, Depaulis A, Deransart C, Piallat B, Marescaux C, Kahane P, Benazzouz A. High-frequency stimulation of the subthalamic nucleus in epilepsy. In: Lüders HO, Comair YG (eds) Epilepsy surgery, 2nd edn. Lippincott-Raven, Philadelphia, pp 821–828
9. Birri R, Perret E, Wieser HG (1982) Der Einfluss verschiedener Temporallappenoperationen auf das Gedächtnis bei Epileptikern. Nervenarzt 53: 144–149
10. Braak E, Olbrich HG, Braak H, Wieser HG, Oertel WH (1986) Glutamic acid decarboxylase immunoreactivity in sector CA1 of the human Ammon's horn. Anat Embryol 175: 15–23
11. Bronen RA, Vives KP, Kim JH, Fulbright RK, Spencer SS, Spencer DD (1997) Focal cortical dysplasia of Taylor, balloon cell subtype: MR differentiation from low-grade tumors. Am J Neuroradiol 18: 1141–1151
12. Buser PA, Talairach J, Bancaud J (1968) Potentiels évoqués, réponses paroxystiques aux stimulations périphériques et zone épileptogène. Rev Neurol 514
13. Buser PA, Bancaud J, Talairach J (1973) Depth recordings in man in temporal lobe epilepsy. In: Brazier MAB (ed) Epilepsy, its phenomena in man. Academic Press, New York, pp 7–97
14. Chelune GJ, Najm IM (2001) Risk factors associated with postsurgical decrements in memory. In: Lüders HO, Comair YG (eds) Epilepsy surgery, 2nd edn. Lippincott-Raven, Philadelphia, pp 497–504
15. Chugani DC, Chugani HT, Muzik O, Shah JR, Shah AK, Canady A, Mangner TJ, Chakraborty PK (1998) Imaging epileptogenic tubers in children with tuberous sclerosis complex using alpha-[11C]methyl-L-tryptophan positron emission tomography. Ann Neurol; 44: 858–866
16. Comte P, Siegfried J, Wieser HG (1983) Multipolar hollow-core electrode for brain recordings. Appl Neurophysiol 46: 41–46
17. Crino PB, Eberwine J (1997) Cellular and molecular basis of cerebral dysgenesis. J Neurosci Res 50: 907–916
18. Crino PB, Duhaime A-C, Baltuch G, White R (2001) Differential expression of glutamate and GABA-A receptor subunit mRNA in cortical dysplasia. Neurology 56: 906–913
19. Cuénod M, Audinat E, Do KQ, Gähwiler BH, Grandes P, Herrling P, Knöpfel T, Perschak H, Streit P, Vollenweider F, Wieser HG (1990) Homocysteic acid as transmitter candidate in the mammalian brain and excitatory amino acids in epilepsy. In: Ben-Ari Y (ed) Excitatory Amino acids and neuronal plasticity. Plenum Press, New York, pp 57–63
20. Dietsch G (1932) Fourier-Analyse von Elektroencephalogramm des Menschen. Pflüger's Arch Ges Physiol 230: 106–112
21. Do KQ, Klancnik J, Gähwiler B, Perschak H, Wieser HG, Cuènod M (1991) Release of excitatory amino acids: animal studies and epileptic foci studies in humans. In: Meldrum BS, Moroni F, Simon RP, Woods JH (eds) Excitatory amino acids. Raven Press Ltd, New York, pp 677–685
22. Dobson J, Grassi PP (1996) Magnetic properties of human hippocampal tissue: evaluation of artefact and contamination sources. Brain Res Bull 39: 255–259
23. Dobson J, Grassi PP (1998) Preliminary evaluation of the magnetic properties of rat brain tissue: implications for models of human interactions with weak electromagnetic fields. J Biochem Molec Biol & Biophys 1: 247–251
24. Dobson JP, Fuller M, Moser S, Wieser HG, Dunn JR, Zoeger J (1995) Evocation of epileptiform activity by weak DC magnetic fields and magnetite biomineralization in the human brain. In: Baumgartner C, Deecke L, Stroink G, Williamson SJ (eds) Biomagnetism: fundamental research and clinical applications. Elsevier/ISO Press, Amsterdam pp 16–19
25. Duc CO, Trabesinger AH, Weber OM, Meier D, Walder M, Wieser HG, Boesiger P (1998) Quantitative 1H-MRS in the evaluation of mesial temporal lobe epilepsy in vivo. Magn Reson Imaging 16: 969–979
26. During MJ, Ryder KM, Spencer DS (1995) Hippocampal GABA transporter function in temporal-lobe epilepsy. Nature 376: 174–177
27. Eder HG, Leber KA, Eustacchio S, Pendl G (2001) The role of gamma knife radiosurgery in children. Childs Nerv Syst 17: 341–347
28. Elger CE, Lehnertz K (1988) Seizure prediction by nonlinear time series analysis of brain electrical activity. Eur J Neurosci 10: 786–789
29. Fandino J, Kollias SS, Wieser HG, Valavanis A, Yonekawa Y (1999) Intraoperative validation of functional magnetic resonance imaging and cortical reorganization patterns in patients with brain tumors involving the primary motor cortex. J Neurosurg 91: 238–250
30. Farrell MA, Droogan O, Secor DL, Poukens V, Quinn B, Vinters HV (1995) Chronic encephalitis associated with epilepsy: immunohistochemical and ultrastructural studies. Acta Neuropathol 89: 313–321
31. Flint AC, Kriegstein AR (1997) Mechanisms underlying neuronal migration disorders and epilepsy. Curr Opin Neurol 10: 92–97
32. Fuller M, Dobson JP, Wieser HG, Moser S (1995) On the sensitivity of the human brain to magnetic fields: Evocation of epileptiform activity. Brain Res Bull 36: 155–159
33. Garcia-Ladona FJ, Palacios JM, Probst A, Wieser HG, Mengod G (1994) Excitatory amino acid AMPA receptor mRNA localization in several regions of normal and neurological disease affected human brain. An in situ hybridization histochemistry study. Molecular Brain Res 21: 75–84
34. Germano IM, Sperber EF (1998) Transplacentally induced neuronal migration disorders: an animal model for the study of the epilepsies. J Neurosci Res 51: 473–488
35. Gotman J (1983) Measurement of small time differences between EEG channels: method and application to epileptic sei-

zure propagation. Electroencephalogr Clin Neurophysiol 56: 501–514
36. Grunwald T, Elger CE, Lehnertz K, Van Roost D, Heinze HJ (1995) Alterations of intrahippocampal cognitive potentials in temporal lobe epilepsy. Electroencephalogr Clin Neurophysiol 95: 53–62
37. Guerrini R, Canapicchi R, Zifkin BG (eds) (1996) Dysplasia of cerebral cortex and epilepsy. Lippincott-Raven, Philadelphia
38. Gundersen V, Danbolt NC, Ottersen OP, Storm-Mathisen J (1993) Demonstration of glutamate/aspartate uptake activity in nerve endings by use of antibodies recognizing exogenous D-aspartate. Neuroscience 57: 97–111
39. Hajek M, Valavanis A, Yonekawa Y, Schiess R, Buck A, Wieser HG (1998) Selective amobarbital test for the determination of language function in patients with epilepsy with frontal and posterior temporal brain lesions. Epilepsia 39: 389–398
40. Halgren E, Squires NK, Wilson CL, Rohrbaugh JW, Babb TL, Crandall PH (1980) Endogenous potentials generated in the human hippocampal formation and amygdala by infrequent events. Science 210: 803–805
41. Halgren E, Baudena P, Clarke JM, Heit G, Liegeois C, Chauvel P, Musolino A (1995a) Intracerebral potentials to rare target and distractor auditory and visual stimuli. I. Superior temporal plane and parietal lobe. Electroencephalogr Clin Neurophysiol 94: 191–220
42. Halgren E, Baudena P, Clakre JM, Heit G, Marinkovic K, Devaux B, Vignal JP, Biraben A (1995b) Intracerebral potentials to rare target and distractor auditory and visual stimuli. II. Medial, lateral and posterior temporal lobe. Electroencephalogr Clin Neurophysiol 94: 229–250
43. Hammers A, Koepp MJ, Richardson MP, Labbé C, Brooks DJ, Cunningham VJ, Duncan JS (2001) Central benzodiazepine receptors in malformations of cortical development: A quantitative study. Brain 124: 1555–1565
44. Hart YM, Cortez M, Andermann F, Hwang P, Fish DR, Dulac O, Silver K, Fejerman N, Cross H, Sherwin A (1994) Medical treatment of Rasmussen's syndrome (chronic encephalitis and epilepsy): effect of high-dose steroids or immunoglobulins in 19 patients. Neurology 44: 1030–1036
45. He XP, Patel M, Whitney KD, Janumpalli S, Tenner A, McNamara JO (1998) Glutamate receptor GluR3 antibodies and death of cortical cells. Neuron 20: 153–163
46. Henke K, Buck A, Weber B, Wieser HG (1997) Human hippocampus establishes associations in memory. Hippocampus 7: 249–256
47. Henke K, Weber B, Kneifel S, Wieser HG, Buck A (1999a) Human hippocampus associates information in memory. Proceedings of the National Academy of Sciences 96: 5884–5889
48. Henke K, Weber B, Schwedler K, Kneifel S, Berthold T, Wieser HG, Buck A (1999b) PET studies of memory. Schweizer Archiv für Neurologie und Psychiatrie 150: 89–96
49. Honavar M, Janota I, Polkey CE (1992) Rasmussen's encephalitis in surgery for epilepsy. Dev Med Child Neurol 34: 3–14
50. Kerfoot C, Vinters HV, Mathern GW (1999) Cerebral cortical dysplasia: giant neurons show potential for incraesed excitation and axonal lasticity. Dev Neurosci 21: 260–270
51. Krauss GL, Campbell ML, Roche KW, Huganir RL, Niedermeyer E (1996) Chronic steroid-responsive encephalitis without autoantibodies to glutamate receptor GluR3. Neurology 46: 247–249
52. Lange HH, Lieb JP, Engel J Jr, Crandall PH (1983) Temporo-spatial patterns of pre-ictal spike activity in human temporal lobe epilepsy. Electroenceph Clin Neurophysiol 56: 543–555
53. Lepage M, Habib R, Tulving E (1998) Hippocampal PET activations of memory encoding and retrieval: the HIPER model. Hippocampus 8: 313–322
54. Lopes da Silva F (1999) EEG analysis: theory and praxis. In: Niedermeyer E, Lopes da Silva F (eds) Electroencephalography: basic principles, clinical applications, and related fields, 4th edn., Williams & Wilkins, Baltimore, pp 1135–1163
55. Loring DW, Meador KJ, King DW, Gallagher BB, Smith JR, Flanigin HF (1988) Relationship of limbic evoked potentials to recent memory performance. Neurology 38: 45–48
56. Loup F, Weinmann O, Yonekawa Y, Aguzzi A, Wieser HG, Fritschy JM (1998) A highly sensitive immunofluorescence procedure for analyzing the subcellular distribution of $GABA_A$ receptor subunits in the human brain. J Histochemistry Cytochemistry 46: 1129–1139
57. Loup F, Wieser HG, Yonekawa Y, Aguzzi A, Fritschy JM (2000) Selective alterations in $GABA_A$ receptor subtypes in human temporal lobe epilepsy. J Neurosci 20: 5401–5419
58. Maton BM, Najm IM, Wang Y, Lüders HO, Ng TC (1999) Postictal in situ MRS brain lactate in the rat kindling model. Neurology 53: 2054–2052
59. McCarthy G, Nobre AC, Bentin S, Spencer DD (1995) Language-related field potentials in the anterior-medial temporal lobe: I. Intracranial distribution and neural generators. J Neurosci 15: 1080–1089
60. McLachlan RS (2001) Vagus nerve stimulation in epilepsy. In: Lüders HO, Comair YG (eds) Epilepsy surgery, 2nd edn. Lippincott-Raven, Philadelphia, pp 813–819
61. Mueller SG, Kollias SS, Trabesinger AH, Buck F, Boesiger P, Wieser HG (2001a) Proton magnetic resonance spectroscopy characteristics of a focal cortical dysgenesis during status epilepticus and in the interictal state. Seizure 10: 518–524
62. Mueller SG, Trabesinger AH, Boesiger P, Wieser HG (2001b) Brain glutathione levels in epileptic patients measured by in vivo 1H-NMR-Spectroscopy. Neurology 57: 1422–1427
63. Mueller SG, Trabesinger AH, Weber OM, Duc CO, Weber B, Meier D, Russ W, Boesiger P, Wieser HG (2001c) Effects of Vigabatrin on brain GABA+/CR signals in epileptics monitored by 1H-NMR-spectroscopy: responder characteristics. Epilepsia 42: 29–40
64. Mueller SG, Weber OM, Boesiger P, Wieser HG (2001d) Influence of pyridoxal 5′-phosphate alone and in combination with vigabatrin on brain GABA measured by 1H-NMR-spectroscopy. Brain Res Bull 55: 555–560
65. Najm IM, Wang Y, Hong SC, Lüders HO, Ng TC, Comair YG (1997) Temporal changes in proton MRS metabolites after kainic acid-induced seizures in rat brain. Epilepsia 38: 87–94
66. Najm IM, Wang Y, Shedid D, Lüders HO, Ng TC, Comair YG (1998) MRS metabolic markers of seizure and seizure-induced neuronal damage. Epilepsia 39: 244–250
67. Nobre AC, Allison T, McCarthy G (1994) Word recognition in the human inferior temporal lobe. Nature 372: 260–263
68. Nobre AC, McCarthy G (1995) Language-related field potentials in the anterior-medial temporal lobe: II. Effects of word type and semantic priming. J Neurosci 15: 1090–1098
69. Oguni H, Andermann F, Rasmussen TB (1991) The natural history of the syndrome of chronic encephalomyelitis and epilepsy: a study of the MNI series of forty-eight cases. In: Andermann F (ed) Chronic encephalitis and epilepsy. Rasmussen's syndrome. Butterworth-Heinemann, Woburn, MA, pp 7–36
70. Paas Y (1998) The pathophysiological mechanism underlying Rasmussen's encephalitis: a debate. TINS 21: 468–469
71. Paller KA, Bozic VS, Ranganath C, Grabowecky M, Yamada S (1999) Brain waves following remembered faces index conscious recollection. Brain Res Cogn Brain Res 7: 519–531

72. Palmini A, Gambardella A, Andermann F, Dubeau F, Da Costa J, Olivier A, Tampieri D, Gloor P, Quesney F, Andermann E, Paglioli E, Paglioli-Neto E, Coutinho L, Leblanc R, Kim HI (1995) Intrinsic epileptogenicity of human dysplastic cortex as suggested by corticography and surgical results. Ann Neurol 37: 476–487
73. Pendl G, Schroettner O, Friehs GM, Feichtinger H (1995) Stereotactic radiosurgery of skull base meningiomas. Stereotact Funct Neurosurg 64 [Suppl] 1: 11–18
74. Pendl G, Eder HG, Schroettner O, Leber KA (1999) Corpus callosotomy with radiosurgery. Neurosurgery 45: 303–308
75. Pendl G, Unger F, Papaefthymiou G, Eustacchio S (2000) Staged radiosurgical treatment for large benign cerebral lesions. J Neurosurg 93 [Suppl] 3: 107–112
76. Pendl G, Eustacchio S, Unger F (2001) Radiosurgery as alternative treatment for skull base meningiomas. J Clin Neurosci 8 [Suppl] 1: 12–14
77. Petroff OAC, Prichard JW, Ogino T, Avison M, Alger JR, Shulman RG (1986) Combined 1H and 31P Nuclear magnetic resonance spectroscopic studies of bicuculline-induced seizures in vivo. Ann Neurol 20: 185–193
78. Petroff OAC, Novotny EJ, Avison M, Rothman DL, Alger JR, Ogino T, Shulman GI, Prichard JW (1992) Cerebral lactate turnover after electroshock: in vivo measurements by 1H/13C magnetic resonance spectroscopy. J Cereb Blood Flow Metab 12: 1022–1029
79. Rasmussen T, Andermann F (1989) Update on the syndrome of "chronic encephalitis" and epilepsy. Cleve Clin J Med [Suppl] 56: 81–84
80. Rasmussen T, Olszweski T, Lloyd-Smith DL (1958) Focal seizures due to chronic localized encephalitis. Neurololy 8: 435–455
81. Régis J, Roberts D (1999) Gamma Knife radiosurgery relative to microsurgery: epilepsy. Stereotact Funct Neurosurg 72 [Suppl] 1: 11–21
82. Régis J, Bartolomei F, Rey M, Genton P, Dravet C, Semah F, Gastaut J, Chauvel P, Peragut J (1999) Gamma knife surgery for mesial temporal lobe epilepsy. Epilepsia 40: 1551–1556
83. Régis J, Bartolomei F, Rey M, Hayashi M, Chauvel P, Peragut JC (2000) Gamma knife surgery for mesial temporal lobe epilepsy. J Neurosurg 93 [Suppl] 3: 3–141
84. Robitaille Y (1991) Neuropathologic aspects of chronic encephalitis. In: Andermann F (ed) Chronic encephalitis and epilepsy. Rasmussen's syndrome. Butterworth-Heinemann, Woburn, MA, pp 79–110
85. Rogers SW, Andrews PI, Gahring LC, Whisenand T, Cauley K, Crain B, Hughes TE, Heinemann SF, McNamara JO (1994) Autoantibodies to glutamate receptor GluR3 in Rasmussen's encephalitis. Science 265: 648–651
86. Roper SN, Gilmore RL, Houser CR (1995) Experimentally induced disorders of neuronal migration produce an increased propensity for electrographic seizures in rats. Epilepsy Res 21: 205–219
87. Sackelares JC, Iasemidis LD, Zaveri HP, Williams WJ (1989) Measurement of chaos to localize seizure onset. Epilepsia 30: 663
88. Sherwin I (1978) Interictal transition in the feline penicillin epileptogenic focus. Electroenceph Clin Neurophysiol 45: 525–534
89. Stapleton JM, Halgren E (1987) Endogenous potentials evoked in simple cognitive tasks: depth components and task correlates. Electroencephalogr Clin Neurophysiol 67: 44–52
90. Stodieck SRG, Wieser HG (1983) The effects of polarization on human epileptic foci. Proceedings First Vienna Workshop on Functional Electrostimulation, abstract, 6 pages
91. Stodieck SRG, Wieser HG (1987) Epicortical DC changes in epileptic patients. In: Wolf P, Dam M, Janz D, Dreifuss FE (eds) Advances in epileptology, vol 16. Raven Press, New York, pp 123–127
92. Strong V, Brown SW, Walker R (1999) Seizure-alert dogs – fact or fiction? Seizure 8: 62–65
93. Tanaka T, Hashizume K, Kunimoto M, Maeda T, Hodozuka A, Nakai H (2001) Multiple subpial transection versus callosal section in the treatment of experimentally induced cortical focal seizures. In: Lüders HO, Comair YG (eds) Epilepsy surgery, 2nd edn. Lippincott-Raven, Philadelphia, pp 801–806
94. Taxt T, Storm-Mathisen J (1984) Uptake of D-aspartate and L-glutamate in excitatory axon terminals in hippocampus: autoradiographic and biochemical comparison with γ-aminobutyrate and other amino acids in normal rats and in rats with lesions. Neurosciene 11: 79–100
95. Taylor DC, Falconer MA, Bruton CJ, Corsellis JA (1971) Focal dysplasia of the cerebral cortex in epilepsy. J Neurol Neurosurg Psychiatry 34: 369–387
96. Tönnes J, Hajek M, Mirkovic N, Stierli B, Behrmann JT, Wieser HG, Streit P (1998) Acute Rasmussen's encephalitis: are there patients without autoantibodies to glutamate receptor GluR3? Society for Neuroscience, Los Angeles
97. Twyman RE, Gahring LC, Spiess J, Rogers SW (1995) Glutamate receptor antibodies activate a subset of receptors and reveal an agonist binding site. Neuron 1995 14: 755–762
98. Velasco M, Velasco F, Velasco AL (1997) Chronic electrical stimulation of the hippocampal formation blocks intractable clinical and EEG temporal lobe epileptogenesis. Paper presented at the 27th Annual Meeting of the Society for Neuroscience. New Orleans, LA, October 25–30, 1997
99. Vinters HV, Emelin JK, Johnson MW, Bushnell T, Kerfoot C (2001) Pathology of cortical dysplasia and malformed brain in neurocutaneous syndromes. In: Lüders HO, Comair YG (eds) Epilepsy surgery, 2nd edn. Lippincott-Raven, Philadelphia, pp 907–914
100. Walsh P (1991) Treatment of Rasmussen's syndrome with intravenous gammaglobulin. In: Andermann F (ed) Chronic encephalitis and epilepsy. Rasmussen's syndrome. Butterworth-Heinemann, Woburn, MA, pp 201–204
101. Wang J, Wieser HG (1994) Regional "rigidity" of background EEG activity in the epileptogenic zone. Epilepsia 1994 35: 495–504
102. Weber B, Lehnertz K, Elger CE, Wieser HG (1998) Neuronal complexity loss in interictal EEG recorded with foramen ovale electrodes predicts side of primary epileptogenic area in temporal lobe epilepsy: a replication study. Epilepsia 39: 922–927
103. Wieser HG (1983) Electroclinical features of the psychomotor seizure. Gustav Fischer-Butterworths, Stuttgart-London
104. Wieser HG (1991) Anterior cerebral artery amobarbital test. In: Lüders HO (ed) Epilepsy surgery. Raven Press, New York, pp 515–523
105. Wieser HG (1998) Electrophysiological aspects of forced normalization. In: Trimble M, Schmitz B (eds) Forced normalization and alternative psychoses of epilepsy. Wrightson Biomedical, U.K. – Petersfield, pp 95–119
106. Wieser HG (1999) EEG, the language of the brain, and its neurochemical souffleuse. Schweiz Arch Neurologie & Psychiatrie 150: 62–71
107. Wieser HG, Yasargil GM (1982) Selective amygdalohippocampectomy as a surgical treatment of mesiobasal limbic epilepsy. Surg Neurol 17: 445–457
108. Wieser HG, Do KQ, Perschak H, Cuénod M (1989) Modulation of extracellular aspartate level during epileptiform events in primary epileptogenic area of patients. Satellite Symposium

of the XXXI Internat. Cong. Physiological Sciences, Helsinki: Physiology, Pharmacology and Development of Epileptogenic Phenomena, July 4–8, 1989, Frankfurt, Abstract

109. Wieser HG, Müller S, Schiess R, Khan N, Regard M, Landis T, Bjeljac M, Buck A, Valavanis A, Yasargil GM, Yonekawa Y (1997) The anterior and posterior selective temporal lobe amobarbital tests: angiographical, clinical, electroencephalographical PET and SPECT findings, and memory performance. Brain Cognition 33: 71–97
110. Wieser HG, Henke K, Zumsteg D, Taub E, Yonekawa Y, Buck A (1999) Activation of left motor cortex during left leg movements following right central resection. J Neurol Neurosurg, Psychiatry 67: 487–491
111. Wieser St (2002) Elektrophysiologische Korrelate der Gedächtnisfunktionen. Thesis, Medical Faculty University Zürich
112. White R, Yue Hua, Scheithauer B, Lynch DR, Henske EP, Crino PB. Selective alterations in glutamate and GABA receptor subunit mRNA expression in dysplastic neurons and giant cells of cortical tubers. Ann Neurol 2001: 49: 67–78
113. Wyler AR (2001) Multiple subpial transections. In: Lüders HO, Comair YG (eds) Epilepsy surgery, 2nd edn. Lippincott-Raven, Philadelphia, pp 807–811
114. Yachnis AT, Powell SZ, Olmsted JJ, Eskin TA (1997) Distinct neurodevelopmental patterns of bcl-2 and bcl-x expression are altered in glioneuronal hamartias of the human temporal lobe. J Neuropathol Exp Neurol 56: 186–198
115. Ying Z, Babb TL, Comair YG, Bingaman W, Bushey M, Touhalisky K (1998) Induced expression of NMDAR2 proteins and differentiated expression of NMDAR1 splice variants in dysplastic neurons of human epileptic neocortex. J Neuropath Exp Neurol 57: 47–62
116. Zhu WJ, Roper SN (2000) Reduced inhibition in an animal model of cortical dysplasia. J Neurosci 20: 8925–8931

Correspondence: Prof. Dr. med. Heinz Gregor Wieser, Abteilung für Epileptologie & Elektroenzephalographie, Neurologische Klinik, Universitätsspital, CH-8091 Zurich.

Acta Neurochir (2002) [Suppl] 84: 17–26

Future Aspects of the Presurgical Evaluation in Epilepsy

M. Feichtinger[1], A. Holl[1], E. Körner[1], O. Schröttner[2], H. Eder[2], F. Unger[2], G. Pendl[2], L. Wurst[3], S. Golaszewski[1], F. Payer[1], F. Fazekas[1], and E. Ott[1]

[1] Department of Neurology, Karl-Franzens University, Graz, Austria
[2] Department of Neurosurgery, Karl-Franzens University, Graz, Austria
[3] Department of Medical Psychology and Psychotherapy, Karl-Franzens University, Graz, Austria

Summary

Epilepsy surgery is a successful therapeutic approach in patients with medically intractable epilepsy. The presurgical evaluation aims to detect the epileptogenic brain area by use of different diagnostic techniques. In this review article the current diagnostic procedures applied for this purpose are described. The diagnostic armamentarium can be divided conceptually into three different groups: assessment of function/dysfunction, structural/morphologic imaging methods and functional neuroimaging techniques. Properties, diagnostic power and limits of all diagnostic tools used in the diagnostic evaluation are discussed. In addition, future perspectives and the diagnostic value of new technologies are mentioned. Some are increasingly gaining acceptance in the routine preoperative diagnostic procedure like MR volumetry or MR spectroscopy of the hippocampus in patients with temporal lobe epilepsy. Some, on the other hand, like MEG and 11C-flumazenil PET, still remain experimental diagnostic tools as they are technically demanding and cost intensive. Besides the refinement of established techniques, co-registration of different modalities like spike-triggered functional MRI will play an important role in the non-invasive detection of the epileptic seizure focus and may change the regimen of the preoperative diagnostic work up of epilepsy patients in the future.

Keywords: Epilepsy surgery; presurgical evaluation; temporal lobe epilepsy; epileptic focus.

Introduction

Within the past decades surgical intervention has become a widely accepted strategy in the therapeutic management of epilepsy. In about 60% of all patients suffering from epilepsy a focally restricted brain area is responsible for the disorder, leading to the diagnosis of focal epilepsy syndromes. Patients with focal epilepsy whose condition can not be adequately controlled with anticonvulsive medication represent potential candidates for surgical epilepsy treatment. Successful surgery depends on the type of focal epilepsy syndrome as well as on the ability to clearly define and sufficiently resect brain regions that are regarded as "epileptogenic". At present about 60% of all patients with focal medically intractable epilepsy operated on remain seizure free after surgery [27].

The principal surgical concept is the complete removal of the "epileptogenic zone" which is defined as brain cortex that is indispensable for the generation of epileptic seizures [55]. Successful epilepsy surgery requires an intensive preoperative diagnostic work-up which should clarify the following items to the epileptologist prior to operation: (i) the accurate localization and extent of the epileptogenic brain area, (ii) exclusion of possible multifocal epileptogenic regions, (iii) preservation of "eloquent" cortex and (iv) evaluation of the individual chance for becoming seizure – free postoperatively. At present, a variety of diagnostic tools are available for answering these questions, such as structural imaging techniques, electrophysiological recordings, neuropsychological testing and functional imaging methods. Considerate interpretation of all these different diagnostic methods is crucial to assess as accurately as possible the patient's individual epileptic condition and the probability of a surgical success. Knowledge about function, the specificity and sensitivity, but also the limits of the different diagnostic methods in defining the epileptogenic area leads to an adequate assessment of each part of the presurgical evaluation.

The fiction of an "ideal presurgical diagnostic tool" could be imaginable as a method defining the epileptogenic brain region with high sensitivity and specificity and in optimal temporal and spatial resolution. This method should favorably be applicable in the interictal state but should reflect the ictal process including its onset. It is unlikely that this ideal presurgical tool for seizure focus determination will ever be available although some of the currently applied tests might offer some of these "ideal" qualities. Electrophysiological recordings such as EEG, for instance, is characterized by a favorable temporal resolution which opened the window for visualizing electric discharges during an epileptic seizure. High resolution MRI techniques, on the other hand, enable the epileptologist to gain detailed insight in the structural integrity or possible pathologic changes of the brain with a considerable spatial resolution. But structural abnormalities need not be epileptogenic per se and brain areas remote from the lesion (e.g. in case of dual pathology) or in the surrounding neighborhood may represent the true epileptogenic region instead [10, 52]. Between these two methodological concepts (functional recording and imaging) a third group of presurgical methods was developed which has been given the term functional neuroimaging. These techniques reflect the aim to make functional ictal phenomena or interictal functional deficits visible in space and to relate them to the epileptogenic zone. Until now, however, methods like interictal SPECT and PET offer only information about dysfunctional areas in the brain (hypoperfusion or hypometabolic) but not on the extent of the epileptogenic region; moreover, the spatial resolution of these techniques is low.

There are two main directions of current research work concerning the different diagnostic methods of the presurgical evaluation: (i) technical improvements to raise the quality of the individual test results and (ii) the combination or co-registration of different methods in order to evaluate whether results of each test may reflect the same neurophysiological or neuropathological process but seen from different points of view. The purpose of this review is to present an overview of possible future developments of the diagnostic tools currently established in the presurgical evaluation of epilepsy patients and to assess whether they may contribute to a better definition of the epileptogenic brain region. According to the different methodological concepts underlying these techniques, the future aspects of the three axes of diagnostic methods are considered separately: the diagnostic axis of function/dysfunction, the diagnostic axis of structural/morphologic imaging and the diagnostic axis of functional neuroimaging. Finally, current and future concepts of co-registration of different methods are listed.

The Diagnostic Axis of Function and Dysfunction

The main concept in this group of diagnostic methods is to evaluate the functional integrity or ictal and interictal functional changes in patients with epilepsy. It is mainly represented by electroencephalographic techniques but also the neurological examination, the analysis of the ictal symptomatology, the neuropsychological assessment of brain dysfunction and finally the recording of electro-magnetic fields (magnetoencephalography) can be included in this diagnostic axis (see Table 1).

Future Aspects of the EEG and ECoG in the Presurgical Evaluation

The development of recording the electrical activity of the human cortex in the first half of the last century offered a completely new understanding of the epileptic condition and the underlying pathophysiological processes during an epileptic seizure. Currently, the simultaneous recording of ictal EEG with the seizure

Table 1. *Evaluation of Functional Features in the Presurgical Evaluation (Diagnostic Axis of Function/Dysfunction)*

Diagnostic methods in clinical use	Experimental diagnostic methods	Future aspects
EEG and ECoG		source dipole models – single dipole modeling – spatio-temporal multiple dipole modeling – realistic headmodel software spike activation use of different anesthetics non-linear analysis – seizure anticipation
Neuropsychological testing		correlation with – MR spectroscopy – MR volumetry – functional MRI
Analysis of seizure symptomatology		analysis of – Vegetative symptoms – Emotional-affective symptoms
	MEG	co-registration with – EEG – realistic head model software – cortical electrical stimulation

EEG Electroencephalography.
ECoG Electrocorticography.
MEG Magneto – encephalography.

symptomatology (video-EEG monitoring) is the gold standard for defining the seizure onset zone in the presurgical work-up. Due to its high temporal resolution not only the seizure onset can accurately be documented but also the propagation of epileptic discharges into other brain areas or into the contralateral hemisphere can eventually be observed. The natural barriers between the brain surface and the electrodes, e.g. the skull, the meninges and the scalp, lead to an attenuated EEG signal, which, in addition, is often distorted by a number of technical and EMG artifacts – especially during an epileptic seizure. A correct localization of the seizure onset zone is often complicated by these limits. Moreover, an estimated area of at least 6 cm^2 of synchronously discharging neurons in the cortex are needed to generate an electric potential that is detectable by surface EEG [16, 22]. Ictal discharges, therefore, may reflect already an electric propagation phenomenon and are not necessarily pointing at the true seizure onset zone. Thus, one aim in the scientific research work is to develop algorithms that enable to define precisely the time of the seizure onset and even to predict a seizure before its clinical manifestation. Anticipation of seizures may be possible by use of nonlinear EEG analysis of intracranial [25] and scalp EEG [63] recordings. Such nonlinear time series analyses would not only contribute to the development of appropriate seizure prevention strategies in the future, they also could improve the diagnostic power of e.g. ictal SPECT studies in the presurgical evaluation.

Beside the ictal EEG analysis interpretation of interictal epileptic activity (spikes) is of high importance for the assessment of postoperative outcome as well as for a precise localization of the irritative zone or the epileptogenic area. Traditional visual EEG inspection is confined to the characterization of the epileptic focus by identifying those electrodes which are recording the maximal negative potential. By use of computer-assisted EEG analysis voltage topography of single spike events or seizure potentials and localization of their source is possible [24]. In recent years different methods for dipole source localization have been developed and were compared with results from intracranial recordings [6, 7]. Although currently not in routine clinical use "single dipole modeling" and "spatio-temporal multiple dipole modeling" will increasingly be an important additional aid for determining the irritative brain area or even the seizure onset zone. Co-registration of dipole modeling data with the individual's MRI will be standard in the next years, as it was shown that by use of realistic head models rather than spherical head models a misplacement of the sources of the dipoles could be reduced to a significant extent [23].

Invasive EEG recordings via subdural stripe and grid electrodes or even intracerebral depth electrodes are part of the preoperative work-up when noninvasive diagnostic tools present inconclusive or divergent results. Their use together with electrical cortical stimulation can also be necessary for the evaluation whether the irritative zone or the seizure onset zone is located within "eloquent" brain regions. In combination, this information can facilitate decisions about the neurosurgical proceeding and the extent of the resection. Intraoperative electrocorticography (ECoG) is also used in many centers to modify the extent of a resection (i.e. "tailored resection") and it may particularly be of value in cases with lesional or MRI negative neocortical epilepsies [61, 77]. Little is known, however, about the influence of anesthetics used during the operation on the ECoG. Several attempts were made to evaluate and compare the frequency and spatial extent of spikes on the ECoG under the use of substances that may activate the neocortex intraoperatively like metohexital [9], propofol [71] or alfentanil [26, 64], but results are inconclusive up to now. Therefore, the primary aim of ongoing research work is to evaluate the influence of different anesthetics on the electrocorticogramm, to assess the optimizied use of anesthetics for the intraoperative definition of localization and extent of the irritative zone and to find the best medical activation method which would allow a reliable resection of primary and secondary epileptogenic brain tissue.

Analysis of Ictal Symptomatology and Neuropsychological Testing

Video analysis of ictal clinical signs is an important part in the presurgical evaluation. A number of studies addressed the frequency as well as the lateralizing and localizing value of different ictal and postictal symptoms such as unilateral ictal dystonia, forced head deviation, ictal speech or postictal dysphasia [5, 20, 41]. Even rare signs as ictal vomiting [4, 13, 18] or ictal urinary urge [3] were reported to serve as lateralizing indicator for the seizure focus. Current and future interests are directed to further clinical signs, that are possibly not as easily detectable but may be also of diagnostic value. Emotional-affective reactions, for instance, like fear, aggression or ecstatic feelings eventually combined with vegetative signs [4] like pallor, rush or mydriasis may point to a seizure onset zone in the non-dominant hemisphere as there is evidence for a hemispheric predominance in the central regulation of autonomic and emotional processes [33]. Some of these symptoms or signs may even serve as indicator for the postoperative outcome as it could be recently shown for the case of ictal fear in temporal lobe epilepsy [28].

Neuropsychological testing is crucial for the detection of discrete functional deficits in a given patient and has gained an indispensable place in the presurgical work-up [50, 57, 67]. There is a high concordance among the epilepsy centers concerning the use of different test modalities. A second important issue is the assessment of postoperative functional deficits – usually by applying the WADA – test. A major interest of the neuropsychological research is to establish non-invasive methods which may replace this invasive procedure in future. MR spectroscopy [62] and functional MRI [36] are new methods that may be of value for assessment of postoperative memory deficits and language representation, respectively, but they still have to be regarded experimental. Another important field of current research work is the role of psychosocial factors for a successful surgical treatment and the optimized postoperative professional care of the patients with epilepsy after surgery [73].

The MEG (Magneto-Encephalography) and its Role in the Presurgical Evaluation

Each epileptiform discharge generates a weak magnetic field, which can be detected by the MEG. Although the sources of EEG and MEG are the same (i.e. neuronal activity), there are major differences between the two measurement quantities [15, 78]. The most important difference is that MEG signals are not subject to distortion by the meninges, the skull or the scalp and that it provides a higher spatial resolution than EEG. On the other hand, MEG can only be studied with patients that are calm and cooperative because MEG detectors need cooling with liquid helium and have to be placed close to the head of the patient due to the weakness of the magnetic potential field. Moreover, different from the EEG, only the tangential part of a current dipole is observable. For the localization of MEG potentials dipole source modeling is applied, preferably with the use of software programs which employ realistic head models instead of spherical models [23]. With this capability to relate epileptic sources to the individual's brain image, MEG provides additional and eventually more precise information than the EEG about the localization of the irritative zone. It can therefore be of complementary diagnostic value in the presurgical evaluation of epilepsy patients. Because of the technical requirements for data acquisition source analysis during seizures using MEG is not possible although there have been reports about ictal recordings of patients [35]. One aim of future research is to develop settings that enable routinely ictal magnetic source imaging. Some efforts have also been made to evaluate the diagnostic power of medical spike activation (e.g. clonidin, metohexital) in order to achieve more reliable data in patients with rare epileptic discharges [38, 39]. Additional scientific research work is directed towards the determination of the spatial relationship between focal epileptic activity and functionally important brain areas [11, 40]. This may reduce the need for invasive ECoG recordings or at least would improve the planning for invasive electrode placement. Although research data are promising MEG is still considered experimental. This may also be due to its high technical demands and its consequently rare availability in only a small number of presurgical epilepsy centers.

The Diagnostic Axis of Structural/Morphologic Imaging

Modern MRI Techniques and their Value for the Definition of the Epileptogenic Lesion

With the application of magnetic resonance imaging to epilepsy, important new insights into the structural basis of temporal lobe epilepsy and into a wide range of other structural abnormalities leading to epileptic seizures have become available (see Table 2). In the presurgical evaluation of epilepsy MRI has, therefore, gained a pivotal role as several cerebral abnormalities like hippocampal sclerosis, small foreign tissue lesions, malformations or cortical developmental abnormalities – all lesions with a high association with the occurrence of epileptic seizures – can be detected with a much higher sensitivity and spatial resolution than before. Thin slice coronal sequences (usually T1-weighted, T2-weighted and fluid attenuation inversion recovery sequences) serve best to detect hippocampal

Table 2. *Imaging Methods in the Presurgical Evaluation – Clinical Use and Experimental Techniques (Diagnostic Axis of Structural Imaging)*

Diagnostic methods in clinical use	Experimental diagnostic methods	Future aspects
Magnetic resonance imaging (MRI) – T2 weighted (coronal) – T1 weighted (coronal, transversal) – FLAIR (fluid attenuated inversion recovery)		
	MR volumetry – hippocampus – amygdala	Correlation with – EEG – histopathological analysis Volumetry of – temporal lobe
	Proton MR spectroscopy – hippocampus	Standardized methodology Value of bilateral pathology Subtle cortical malformations 31 P MR spectroscopy
	Perfusion MRI	Diagnostic value? Correlation with – SPECT
	Diffusion MRI	Diagnostic value? – complex partial seizures – secondary generalized seizures Postictal diffusion MRI

31 P MR spectroscopy = 31 Phosphorous magnetic resonance spectroscopy.
EEG Electroencephalography.
SPECT Single photon emission computed tomography.

sclerosis and contrast enhanced scans may be necessary to define malignant lesions. The detection of cortical dysgenesis, a frequent cause of medically intractable epilepsy [53, 69], is also an important issue. These often very subtle cerebral abnormalities are commonly not visible on routine MRI sequences. There is evidence that dysplastic cortical changes may extend beyond the visible lesion and thus are likely to account for some of the less successful outcomes after surgical treatment [53, 70]. Several technical attempts like the use of surface coils [31], automated segmentation and quantification of cerebral gray matter [65, 79] or curvilinear reformatting [2] were reported to be helpful in detecting subtle cortical malformations when routine MRI was negative. However, whether these technical improvements will serve as a reliable tool in the clinical practice of presurgical work-up remains to be clarified.

Two MRI technologies established in recent years are also gaining increasingly clinical acceptance, both attempting to detect hippocampal sclerosis preoperatively: the volumetric measurement of the hippocampus and proton MR spectroscopy. Hippocampal volume (including the amygdala) can best be determined from 3D data sets; unilateral or bilateral atrophy of these brain structures (indicating possible sclerosis) can be assessed after correction with the total brain volume and in comparison with normal controls [47]. Whether significantly smaller volumes of different other brain regions, e.g. of the entire temporal lobes, are indicative of lateralizing the epileptogenic area is not known although there are reports about a relation between temporal lobe epilepsy and unilateral atrophy of the whole temporal lobe [48].

Proton MR spectroscopy can also serve to indicate pathology as N-acetyl-aspartate (NAA) is considered to be a neuronal marker and reduction of NAA is likely to indicate the loss or dysfunction of neurons. The decrease of NAA is determined either by calculation of the NAA/choline or NAA/creatin ratio but recently can also be quantified in absolute terms. Proton MR spectroscopy serves as a reliable additional indicator for (unilateral or bilateral) hippocampal sclerosis or dysfunction in the presurgical diagnostic evaluation. There are two methodologies currently used: single voxel MR spectroscopy which assesses larger brain volumes and multivoxel chemical shift imaging (CSI) which, though subject to a higher risk for artifacts, offers the opportunity to investigate multiple small voxels throughout larger areas of the brain [12, 51]. Goals of the future research work concerning this technique are (i) to evaluate the prognostic value of bilateral hippocampal metabolic changes for the postoperative outcome [21], (ii) to establish a standardized methodology which is available in the clinical practice (iii) to assess whether proton chemical shift imaging may add information regarding subtle, more widespread developmental disorders of the cortex which extend beyond the MRI visible lesion and (iv) to evaluate the diagnostic contribution of other MR spectroscopic technologies like the 31P-spectroscopy for the presurgical evaluation [45].

Several other MRI based techniques merit to be mentioned although their value for the clinical use has still to be elucidated in the future: there is some evidence that measuring the apparent diffusion coefficient (ADC) interictally is also indicative of hippocampal sclerosis [34]. Diffusion MRI may be especially useful after status epilepticus or after a series of seizures in order to detect the seizure focus [14, 19, 37]. If postictal studies after complex partial seizures provide sufficient information to outline the seizure onset zone is currently under discussion. Although magnetization transfer imaging recently was shown not to be able to reliably detect hippocampal sclerosis [54, 75], perfusion MRI might be an additional tool for showing subtle hypoperfusion within possibly dysfunctional brain regions [66, 80]. The importance of these two techniques for the preoperative diagnosis, however, is not clear yet.

In conclusion MRI offers a variety of different methoodologies that can be of use in the presurgical work-up of epilepsy surgery candidates. Many of these techniques have to be considered still experimental and are in the stage of research work at present but due to the continuous evolution of MRI technology, some may soon become accepted tools in the diagnostic armamentarium of the epileptologist.

The Diagnostic Axis of Functional Neuroimaging

An epileptic focus can be interpreted as a brain area which is – ictally or interictally – different from the surrounding brain with respect to various functional properties. Based on this concept functional neuroimaging technologies like single photon emisssion computed tomography (SPECT) and positron emission tomography (PET) aim to visualize these functional changes, to relate them either to the epileptogenic zone or the seizure onset zone and to evaluate the extent of these zones within the brain. It is current standard to use interictal and ictal SPECT and [18F]fluorodeoxyglucose-PET (FDG-PET) in the evaluation of epilepsy surgery candidates (see Table 3).

Table 3. *Functional Neuroimaging Techniques in the Presurgical Evaluation (Diagnostic Axis of Functional Neuroimaging)*

Diagnostic methods in clinical use	Experimental diagnostic methods	Future aspects
SPECT – Interictal – Ictal – Subtracted ictal SPECT co-registrated with MRI (SISCOM)		Seizure anticipation technology + ictal SPECT Technical refinement
PET – FDG-PET	– Flumazenil PET – Opioid-Receptor PET – L-Tryptophan PET	Neurotransmitter PET Correlation with – EEG – FDG-PET – SPECT
Functional MRI – Language mapping – Somatosensory mapping	– Spike-triggered functional MRI	Memory function Correlation with – electro-cortical stimulation – PET – WADA Test Correlation with dipole models – MEG – SPECT – PET

SPECT Single photon emission computed tomography.
PET Positron emission tomography.
FDG-PET 18 Fluorodeoxyglucose-PET.
MRI Magnetic resonance imaging.
MEG Magneto-encephalography.

Interictal SPECT, Ictal SPECT and Subtraction Ictal SPECT co-Registered to MRI (SISCOM)

The use of radiotracers such as technetium 99m-ethyl-cysteinate-dimer (ECD) or technetium-99m-hexamethylpropylene-amine-oxime (HMPAO) provide a semiquantitative image of cerebral blood flow within 30–60 s after injection. This can be used for both interictal and ictal SPECT studies. Interictal SPECT usually displays the epileptogenic region as an area of hypoperfusion. In the ictal state an epileptic seizure focus is associated with local hyperperfusion. Whereas interictal SPECT repeatedly showed disappointing results concerning sensitivity for the localization of an epileptic focus, ictal SPECT is regarded as highly specific and sensitive for determination of the seizure onset zone [72, 76]. The estimated sensitivity of ictal SPECT in temporal lobe epilepsy is approximately 75–90% and somewhat lower in extratemporal epilepsy (~60%) – probably due to a more rapid spread of epileptic discharges to other brain regions [56, 72, 81]. Further improvements of the sensitivity can be achieved by a comparison and subtraction of ictal and interictal SPECT scans after they have been co-registered with the patient's MRI (SISCOM) [58, 59]. Future clinical research concerning the measurement of cerebral blood flow with SPECT technology will have to include the relationship between electrophysiological data (EEG, MEG, dipole models) and results obtained from ictal and interictal SPECT studies.

FDG-PET and Related Future Technologies

PET has been used for the evaluation of seizures and focal dysfunctional brain regions by an increasing number of centers in the last years. FDG-PET scans reflect cerebral metabolic rates for glucose over a 5–10 minute uptake period. About 70–80% of patients with "localization-related epilepsy" – complex partial and secondary generalized seizures – have interictal focal hypometabolism on FDG-PET [1, 74] compatible with the epileptic focus as determined by EEG. PET hypometabolism, however, is frequently more extensive than the abnormalities detected on MRI, probably due to distant metabolic suppression from the structural lesion [1, 74]. FDG-PET is currently in use in the presurgical work-up as complementary diagnostic tool but can only be applied interictally.

Flumazenil is a specific, reversibly bound central benzodiazepine receptor antagonist, and 11C-flumazenil is a PET-ligand that acts as a useful marker of the binding of gamma-amino-butyric acid to central benzodiazepine receptors [60]. 11C-flumazenil PET showed reduced binding of this ligand to central benzodiazepine receptors in epileptogenic foci [68]. Compared to measurements of the cerebral metabolic rate for glucose via FDG-PET, 11C-flumazenil PET seems to be more precise in circumscribing the site of the epileptic focus. Future studies are needed, however, to identify if there are subgroups of patients where one tracer is preferable to the other and whether benzodiazepine receptor labeled PET scans may be also of value in extratemporal epilepsies. More recently, PET scans using opioid receptor ligands (11C-carfentanil, 11C-diprenorphine) provided a similar sensitivity concerning the seizure lateralization as FDG-PET [29]. Along with the increasing knowledge about the role of neurotransmitter and receptor physiology and the neurophysiological processes during an epileptic seizure, several neurotransmitter and receptor PET technologies will be available and studied in the future. This may allow to obtain images of differences in neurotransmitter distribution which could lead to a better interpretation of epileptogenicity and may guide the surgical resection in a much more accurate manner than it is possible today.

The Functional MRI – The Missing Link Between Function and Image?

With the use of blood oxygenation level-dependent (BOLD) functional MRI (fMRI) vascular response to circumscribed neural activity can be measured. This technique, therefore, provides information about the functional status of small brain areas that are activated by various paradigms e.g. somatosensory stimuli or active movements. This method is also of clinical importance and will increasingly be in the future – for speech lateralization and detection of "eloquent" cortex in the course of the presurgical evaluation and the preoperative determination of the extent of brain cortex that can be resected without significant deficits [17, 30]. To date, intracarotid amobarbital testing (WADA test) remains the "gold standard" to evaluate language representation and memory function before planning surgery. There have been promising reports about mapping language functions by use of fMRI [8] which give hope that the WADA test could be replaced by this non-invasive technique in the near future. Concerning the memory function of the hippocampus, however, few convincing results are available which demonstrate that fMRI could be also used for assessing these functions [32, 36].

Resection close to functionally important brain regions requires exact knowledge of the individual mapping of somatosensory, motor or higher-level cognitive brain functions. Using electrocorticography and stimulation techniques pre- and intraoperatively, an optimized guidance for the neurosurgeon can be offered. Functional MRI is capable of detecting very small areas of focal brain activation and represents therefore a non-invasive alternative to electrostimulation studies in the preoperative evaluation [44]. Although serial studies comparing both investigative procedures are lacking, functional MRI is nonetheless a very promising technique that may dramatically change the presurgical diagnostic regimen in epilepsy patients in the near future.

Epileptic activity in form of electric discharges – be it a single spike or an epileptic seizure – leads to a reactive increase in blood flow as a direct response to the hyperactivity of the respective neuronal population. Spike-triggered fMRI aims to detect focal activation of single epileptic discharges and to relate them to the coregistered magnetic resonance image of the patient [42, 43, 49]. These studies are part of current intensive research and first results on revealing irritative brain areas in this manner have already been reported. The use of fMRI for defining the seizure onset zone, however, is limited to patients with seizures of short duration or without motor symptoms and will therefore not be regularly applicable in clinical practice.

In conclusion, the major benefits of fMRI for the presurgical evaluation will probably be found in the non-invasive determination of memory and language function, the preoperative mapping of brain functions and the interpretation of epileptiform discharges with respect to the irritative zone within the epileptic brain.

Conclusion – The Diagnostic Network

Besides the technical refinements of all diagnostic tools that are employed for seizure focus localization, there is a large interest in the current scientific research to compare the different techniques with one another in order to evaluate their clinical value and to underpin their sensitivity and specificity. This is performed by co-registration of functional methods with morphological imaging or functional imaging technologies. Of special diagnostic power in the presurgical work-up will be the subtraction of ictal and interictal SPECT scans co-registrated with the MRI (SISCOM) technique [58, 59], the spike-triggered functional MRI [42, 43, 49] and co-registration of electroencephalographic data (dipole source models), or magnetoencephalographic with tomographic imaging methods (MRI, PET). This comparative research will undoubtedly lead to a significant change in the presurgical work-up as invasive EEG recordings may become more and more dispensable by the use of these reliable non-invasive diagnostic methods in the future.

All scientific attempts are directed towards a correct and reliable detection of the epileptogenic zone which includes the commonly called "epileptic focus". None of the currently available diagnostic concepts permits a direct measurement of the epileptogenic zone that is per definition the brain cortex which generates the epileptic seizures. The search for new techniques defining accurately this epileptogenic area is especially encouraging in the field of receptor PET studies, which will lead also to a better understanding of the neuropathological processes in the course of an epileptic seizure. Besides resective surgery, concepts of radiosurgery are currently under investigation – non-invasive presurgical diagnosis will play an even more important role for patients undergoing this therapy in the future. Seizure anticipation may perhaps be of utmost importance when palliative surgical treatment, for instance local application of benzodiazepines on the seizure onset zone using small implanted pumps, will be a serious therapeutic alternative.

Considering the high percentages of average seizure free rates, reported by many centers, epilepsy surgery must be regarded as a very successful therapeutic concept in medically intractable epilepsy patients. An intensive and accurate presurgical diagnostic evaluation for seizure focus localization and for assessment of possible postoperative functional deficits is indispensable for a successful surgical intervention. Refinements of current and development of future diagnostic tools as well as the co-registration of established technologies are the principal concepts with which an increasing diagnostic power in the presurgical evaluation can be expected in the future.

References

1. Abou-Khalil BW, Siegel GJ, Sackellares JC, Gilman S, Hichwa R, Marshall R (1987) Positron emission tomography studies of cerebral glucose metabolism in chronic partial epilepsy. Ann Neurol 22: 480–486
2. Bastos AC, Comeau RM, Andermann F, Melanson D, Cendes F, Dubeau F, Fontaine S, Tampieri D, Olivier A (1999) Diagnosis of subtle focal dysplastic lesions: curvilinear reformatting from three-dimensional magnetic resonance imaging. Ann Neurol 46: 88–94
3. Baumgartner C, Groppel G, Leutmezer F, Aull-Watschinger S, Pataraia E, Feucht M, Trinka E, Unterberger I, Bauer G (2000) Ictal urinary urge indicates seizure onset in the nondominant temporal lobe. Neurology 55: 432–434
4. Baumgartner C, Lurger S, Leutmezer F (2001) Autonomic symptoms during epileptic seizures. Epileptic Disord 3: 103–116
5. Bleasel A, Kotagal P, Kankirawatana P, Rybicki L (1997) Lateralizing value and semiology of ictal limb posturing and version in temporal lobe and extratemporal epilepsy. Epilepsia 38: 168–174
6. Boon P, D'Have M, Van HG, Vanrumste B, Vonck K, Adam C, Vandekerckhove T, Michielsen G, Baulac M, De RJ (1999) Source localization in refractory partial epilepsy. Rev Neurol (Paris) 155: 499–508
7. Boon P, D'Have M, Vandekerckhove T, Achten E, Adam C, Clemenceau S, Baulac M, Goossens L, Calliauw L, De RJ (1997) Dipole modelling and intracranial EEG recording: correlation between dipole and ictal onset zone. Acta Neurochir (Wien) 139: 643–652
8. Carpentier A, Pugh KR, Westerveld M, Studholme C, Skrinjar O, Thompson JL, Spencer DD, Constable RT (2001) Functional MRI of language processing: dependence on input modality and temporal lobe epilepsy. Epilepsia 42: 1241–1254
9. Cascino GD, So EL, Sharbrough FW, Strelow D, Lagerlund TD, Milde LN, O'Brien PC (1993) Alfentanil-induced epileptiform activity in patients with partial epilepsy. J Clin Neurophysiol 10: 520–525
10. Cascino G, Boon P, Fish D (1993) Surgically remediable lesional syndromes. In: Engel J (ed) Surgical treatment of the epilepsies. Raven Press, New York
11. Castillo EM, Simos PG, Venkataraman V, Breier JI, Wheless JW, Papanicolaou AC (2001) Mapping of expressive language cortex using magnetic source imaging. Neurocase 7: 419–422
12. Cendes F, Caramanos Z, Andermann F, Dubeau F, Arnold DL (1997) Proton magnetic resonance spectroscopic imaging and magnetic resonance imaging volumetry in the lateralization of

temporal lobe epilepsy: a series of 100 patients. Ann Neurol 42: 737–746
13. Chen C, Yen DJ, Yiu CH, Shih YH, Yu HY, Su MS (1999) Ictal vomiting in partial seizures of temporal lobe origin. Eur Neurol 42: 235–239
14. Chu K, Kang DW, Kim JY, Chang KH, Lee SK (2001) Diffusion-weighted magnetic resonance imaging in nonconvulsive status epilepticus. Arch Neurol 58: 993–998
15. Cohen D, Cuffin BN, Yunokuchi K, Maniewski R, Purcell C, Cosgrove GR, Ives J, Kennedy JG, Schomer DL (1990) MEG versus EEG localization test using implanted sources in the human brain. Ann Neurol 28: 811–817
16. Cooper R, Winter A, Crow H, Walter W (1965) Comparison of subcortical, cortical and scalp activity using chronically indwelling electrodes in man. Electroencephalogr Clin Neurophysiol 18: 217–228
17. Detre JA, Floyd TF (2001) Functional MRI and its applications to the clinical neurosciences. Neuroscientist 7: 64–79
18. Devinsky O, Frasca J, Pacia SV, Luciano DJ, Paraiso J, Doyle W (1995) Ictus emeticus: further evidence of nondominant temporal involvement. Neurology 45: 1158–1160
19. Diehl B, Najm I, Ruggieri P, Tkach J, Mohamed A, Morris H, Wyllie E, Fisher E, Duda J, Lieber M, Bingaman W, Luders HO (2001) Postictal diffusion-weighted imaging for the localization of focal epileptic areas in temporal lobe epilepsy. Epilepsia 42: 21–28
20. Dupont S, Semah F, Boon P, Saint-Hilaire JM, Adam C, Broglin D, Baulac M (1999) Association of ipsilateral motor automatisms and contralateral dystonic posturing: a clinical feature differentiating medial from neocortical temporal lobe epilepsy. Arch Neurol 56: 927–932
21. Eberhardt KE, Stefan H, Buchfelder M, Pauli E, Hopp P, Huk W, Tomandl BF (2000) The significance of bilateral CSI changes for the postoperative outcome in temporal lobe epilepsy. J Comput Assist Tomogr 24: 919–926
22. Ebersole JS (1997) Defining epileptogenic foci: past, present, future. J Clin Neurophysiol 14: 470–483
23. Ebersole JS (2000) Noninvasive localization of epileptogenic foci by EEG source modeling. Epilepsia 41 [Suppl] 3: S24–S33
24. Ebersole JS, Wade PB (1991) Spike voltage topography identifies two types of frontotemporal epileptic foci. Neurology 41: 1425–1433
25. Elger CE, Widman G, Andrzejak R, Arnhold J, David P, Lehnertz K (2001) Nonlinear EEG analysis and its potential role in epileptology. Epilepsia 41 [Suppl] 3: S34–S38
26. Endo T, Sato K, Shamoto H, Yoshimoto T (2002) Effects of sevoflurane on electrocorticography in patients with intractable temporal lobe epilepsy. J Neurosurg Anesthesiol 14: 59–62
27. Engel JJ (1993) Update on surgical treatment of the epilepsies. Summary of the Second International Palm Desert Conference on the Surgical Treatment of the Epilepsies (1992). Neurology 43: 1612–1617
28. Feichtinger M, Pauli E, Schafer I, Eberhardt KW, Tomandl B, Huk J, Stefan H (2001) Ictal fear in temporal lobe epilepsy: surgical outcome and focal hippocampal changes revealed by proton magnetic resonance spectroscopy imaging. Arch Neurol 58: 771–777
29. Frost JJ, Mayberg HS, Fisher RS, Douglass KH, Dannals RF, Links JM, Wilson AA, Ravert HT, Rosenbaum AE, Snyder SH (1988) Mu-opiate receptors measured by positron emission tomography are increased in temporal lobe epilepsy. Ann Neurol 23: 231–237
30. Gaillard WD, Bookheimer SY, Cohen M (2000) The use of fMRI in neocortical epilepsy. Adv Neurol 84: 391–404
31. Grant PE, Barkovich AJ, Wald LL, Dillon WP, Laxer KD, Vigneron DB (1997) High-resolution surface-coil MR of cortical lesions in medically refractory epilepsy: a prospective study. AJNR 18: 291–301
32. Hammeke TA, Bellgowan PS, Binder JR (2000) fMRI: methodology-cognitive function mapping. Adv Neurol 83: 221–233
33. Hilz MJ, Dutsch M, Perrine K, Nelson PK, Rauhut U, Devinsky O (2001) Hemispheric influence on autonomic modulation and baroreflex sensitivity. Ann Neurol 49: 575–584
34. Hugg JW, Butterworth EJ, Kuzniecky RI (1999) Diffusion mapping applied to mesial temporal lobe epilepsy: preliminary observations. Neurology 53: 173–176
35. Ishibashi H, Morioka T, Shigeto H, Nishio S, Yamamoto T, Fukui M (1998) Three-dimensional localization of subclinical ictal activity by magnetoencephalography: correlation with invasive monitoring. Surg Neurol 50: 157–163
36. Jokeit H, Okujava M, Woermann FG (2001) Memory fMRI lateralizes temporal lobe epilepsy. Neurology 57: 1786–1793
37. Kim JA, Chung JI, Yoon PH, Kim DI, Chung TS, Kim EJ, Jeong EK (2001) Transient MR signal changes in patients with generalized tonicoclonic seizure or status epilepticus: periictal diffusion-weighted imaging. AJNR 22: 1149–1160
38. Kirchberger K, Schmitt H, Hummel C, Peinemann A, Pauli E, Kettenmann B, Stefan H (1998a) Clonidine- and methohexital-induced epileptiform discharges detected by magnetoencephalography (MEG) in patients with localization-related epilepsies. Epilepsia 39: 1104–1112
39. Kirchberger K, Schmitt H, Hummel C, Peinemann A, Pauli E, Kettenmann B, Stefan H (1998b) Clonidine and methohexital-induced epileptic magnetoencephalographic discharges in patients with focal epilepsies. Epilepsia 39: 841–849
40. Kober H, Nimsky C, Moller M, Hastreiter P, Fahlbusch R, Ganslandt O (2001) Correlation of sensorimotor activation with functional magnetic resonance imaging and magnetoencephalography in presurgical functional imaging: a spatial analysis. Neuroimage 14: 1214–1228
41. Kotagal P (1999) Significance of dystonic posturing with unilateral automatisms. Arch Neurol 56: 912–913
42. Krakow K, Lemieux L, Messina D, Scott CA, Symms MR, Duncan JS, Fish DR (2001) Spatio-temporal imaging of focal interictal epileptiform activity using EEG-triggered functional MRI. Epileptic Disord 3: 67–74
43. Krakow K, Woermann FG, Symms MR, Allen PJ, Lemieux L, Barker GJ, Duncan JS, Fish DR (1999) EEG-triggered functional MRI of interictal epileptiform activity in patients with partial seizures. Brain 122: 1679–1688
44. Kurth R, Villringer K, Mackert BM, Schwiemann J, Braun J, Curio G, Villringer A, Wolf KJ (1998) fMRI assessment of somatotopy in human Brodmann area 3b by electrical finger stimulation. Neuroreport 9: 207–212
45. Kuzniecky R (1999) Magnetic resonance spectroscopy in focal epilepsy: 31P and 1H spectroscopy. Rev Neurol (Paris) 155: 495–498
46. Kuzniecky R, Hugg J, Hetherington H, Martin R, Faught E, Morawetz R, Gilliam F (1999) Predictive value of 1H MRSI for outcome in temporal lobectomy. Neurology 53: 694–698
47. Kuzniecky RI, Bilir E, Gilliam F, Faught E, Palmer C, Morawetz R, Jackson G (1997) Multimodality MRI in mesial temporal sclerosis: relative sensitivity and specificity. Neurology 49: 774–778
48. Lee JW, Reutens DC, Dubeau F, Evans A, Andermann F (1995) Morphometry in temporal lobe epilepsy. Magn Reson Imaging 13: 1073–1080

49. Lemieux L, Krakow K, Fish DR (2001) Comparison of spike-triggered functional MRI BOLD activation and EEG dipole model localization. Neuroimage 14: 1097–1104
50. Lezak MD (1983) Neuropsychological assessment. Oxford University Press, New York
51. Li LM, Cendes F, Andermann F, Dubeau F, Arnold DL (2000) Spatial extent of neuronal metabolic dysfunction measured by proton MR spectroscopic imaging in patients with localization-related epilepsy. Epilepsia 41: 666–674
52. Li LM, Cendes F, Watson C, Andermann F, Fish DR, Dubeau F, Free S, Olivier A, Harkness W, Thomas DG, Duncan JS, Sander JW, Shorvon SD, Cook MJ, Arnold DL (1997) Surgical treatment of patients with single and dual pathology: relevance of lesion and of hippocampal atrophy to seizure outcome. Neurology 48: 437–444
53. Li LM, Fish DR, Sisodiya SM, Shorvon SD, Alsanjari N, Stevens JM (1995) High resolution magnetic resonance imaging in adults with partial or secondary generalised epilepsy attending a tertiary referral unit. J Neurol Neurosurg Psychiatry 59: 384–387
54. Li LM, Narayanan S, Pike GB, Andermann F, Dubeau F, Arnold DL (2000) Magnetization transfer ratio is unable to lateralize epileptic foci in patients with temporal lobe epilepsy. AJNR 21: 1853–1856
55. Lüders H, Awad I (1992) Conceptual considerations. In: Luders HO (ed) Epilepsy surgery. Raven Press, New York
56. Markand ON, Salanova V, Worth R, Park HM, Wellman HN (1997) Comparative study of interictal PET and ictal SPECT in complex partial seizures. Acta Neurol Scand 95: 129–136
57. Milner B (1975) Psychological aspects of focal epilepsy and its neurosurgical management. Adv Neurol 8: 299–321
58. O'Brien TJ, So EL, Mullan BP, Cascino GD, Hauser MF, Brinkmann BH, Sharbrough FW, Meyer FB (2000) Subtraction peri-ictal SPECT is predictive of extratemporal epilepsy surgery outcome. Neurology 55: 1668–1677
59. O'Brien TJ, So EL, Mullan BP, Hauser MF, Brinkmann BH, Bohnen NI, Hanson D, Cascino GD, Jack CRJ, Sharbrough FW (1998) Subtraction ictal SPECT co-registered to MRI improves clinical usefulness of SPECT in localizing the surgical seizure focus. Neurology 50: 445–454
60. Olsen RW, McCabe RT, Wamsley JK (1990) GABAA receptor subtypes: autoradiographic comparison of GABA, benzodiazepine, and convulsant binding sites in the rat central nervous system. J Chem Neuroanat 3: 59–76
61. Palmini A, Gambardella A, Andermann F, Dubeau F, da CJ, Olivier A, Tampieri D, Gloor P, Quesney F, Andermann E (1995) Intrinsic epileptogenicity of human dysplastic cortex as suggested by corticography and surgical results. Ann Neurol 37: 476–487
62. Pauli E, Eberhardt KW, Schafer I, Tomandl B, Huk WJ, Stefan H (2000) Chemical shift imaging spectroscopy and memory function in temporal lobe epilepsy. Epilepsia 41: 282–289
63. Protopopescu VA, Hively AL, Gailey PC (2001) Epileptic event forewarning from scalp EEG. J Clin Neurophysiol 18: 223–245
64. Ragazzo PC, Galanopoulou AS (2000) Alfentanil-induced activation: a promising tool in the presurgical evaluation of temporal lobe epilepsy patients. Brain Res Brain Res Rev 32: 316–327
65. Richardson MP, Friston KJ, Sisodiya SM, Koepp MJ, Ashburner J, Free SL, Brooks DJ, Duncan JS (1997) Cortical grey matter and benzodiazepine receptors in malformations of cortical development. A voxel-based comparison of structural and functional imaging data. Brain 120: 1961–1973
66. Sagiuchi T, Ishii K, Asano Y, Aoki Y, Woodhams R, Yanaihara H, Kan S, Hayakawa K (2001) Transient seizure activity demonstrated by Tc-99 m HMPAO SPECT and diffusion-weighted MR imaging. Ann Nucl Med 15: 267–270
67. Sass KJ, Spencer DD, Kim JH, Westerveld M, Novelly RA, Lencz T (1990) Verbal memory impairment correlates with hippocampal pyramidal cell density. Neurology 40: 1694–1697
68. Savic I, Persson A, Roland P, Pauli S, Sedvall G, Widen L (1988) In-vivo demonstration of reduced benzodiazepine receptor binding in human epileptic foci. Lancet 2: 863–866
69. Semah F, Picot MC, Adam C, Broglin D, Arzimanoglou A, Bazin B, Cavalcanti D, Baulac M (1998) Is the underlying cause of epilepsy a major prognostic factor for recurrence? Neurology 51: 1256–1262
70. Sisodiya SM (2000) Surgery for malformations of cortical development causing epilepsy. Brain 123: 1075–1091
71. Soriano SG, Eldredge EA, Wang FK, Kull L, Madsen JR, Black PM, Riviello JJ, Rockoff MA (2000) The effect of propofol on intraoperative electrocorticography and cortical stimulation during awake craniotomies in children. Paediatr Anaesth 10: 29–34
72. Stefan H, Hopp P, Platsch G, Kuwert T (2000) SPECT: ictal perfusion in localization-related epilepsies. Adv Neurol 83: 41–50
73. Suurmeijer TP, Reuvekamp MF, Aldenkamp BP (2001) Social functioning, psychological functioning, and quality of life in epilepsy. Epilepsia 42: 1160–1168
74. Theodore WH, Newmark ME, Sato S, Brooks R, Patronas N, De LP, DiChiro G, Kessler RM, Margolin R, Manning RG (1983) [18F]fluorodeoxyglucose positron emission tomography in refractory complex partial seizures. Ann Neurol 14: 429–437
75. Tofts PS, Sisodiya S, Barker GJ, Webb S, MacManus D, Fish F, Shorvon S (1995) MR magnetization transfer measurements in temporal lobe epilepsy: a preliminary study. AJNR 16: 1862–1863
76. Weil S, Noachtar S, Arnold S, Yousry TA, Winkler PA, Tatsch K (2001) Ictal ECD-SPECT differentiates between temporal and extratemporal epilepsy: confirmation by excellent postoperative seizure control. Nucl Med Commun 22: 233–237
77. Wennberg R, Quesney F, Olivier A, Rasmussen T (1998) Electrocorticography and outcome in frontal lobe epilepsy. Electroencephalogr Clin Neurophysiol 106: 357–368
78. Williamson SJ, Lu ZL, Karron D, Kaufman L (1991) Advantages and limitations of magnetic source imaging. Brain Topogr 4: 169–180
79. Woermann FG, Free SL, Koepp MJ, Ashburner J, Duncan JS (1999) Voxel-by-voxel comparison of automatically segmented cerebral gray matter – A rater-independent comparison of structural MRI in patients with epilepsy. Neuroimage 10: 373–384
80. Wolf RL, Alsop DC, Levy-Reis I, Meyer PT, Maldjian JA, Gonzalez-Atavales J, French JA, Alavi A, Detre JA (2001) Detection of mesial temporal lobe hypoperfusion in patients with temporal lobe epilepsy by use of arterial spin labeled perfusion MR imaging. AJNR 22: 1334–1341
81. Won HJ, Chang KH, Cheon JE, Kim HD, Lee DS, Han MH, Kim IO, Lee SK, Chung CK (1999) Comparison of MR imaging with PET and ictal SPECT in 118 patients with intractable epilepsy. AJNR Am J Neuroradiol 20: 593–599

Correspondence: Feichtinger Michael, M.D., Department of Neurology, Karl-Franzens University, Auenbruggerplatz 22, A-8036 Graz, Austria.

Acta Neurochir (2002) [Suppl] 84: 27–35

Surgical Treatment of Epilepsies

J. Zentner

Department of Neurosurgery, University of Freiburg, Freiburg, Germany

Summary

Epilepsy is characterized by recurrent epileptic seizures. Surgical interventions represent a reasonable alternative to long-term anti-epileptic drug treatment in those patients destined to achieve incomplete seizure control. The presurgical work-up aims at identifying appropriate surgical candidates. Surgical options with a curative goal include temporal and extratemporal resections and hemispherectomy. With these procedures complete seizure control can be achieved in approximately 2/3 of patients. With palliative procedures such as callosotomy, multiple subpial transections, and vagal nerve stimulation, approximately half of the patients will significantly improve after surgery. In all, epilepsy surgery has proven to be a highly effective treatment option. Major problems include the definition of the epileptogenic area with respect to optimal seizure control and minimum neurological and neuropsychological impairment after surgery.

Keywords: Epilepsy; surgical treatment; medical treatment.

Historical Background

In Europe, epilepsy surgery began in 1886, when Victor Horsley resected a scar of the motor cortex in a 22-year old patient suffering from focal motor seizures that had been caused 15 years earlier by a depressed fracture [10]. In Germany, surgeons like Fedor Krause of Berlin extended the indication for epilepsy surgery to other etiologies [11]. Together with his coworker Schum, Krause dedicated one volume of his work "Die spezielle Chirurgie der Gehirnkrankheiten" to epilepsies. In this monograph he discussed interventions like lumbar puncture, pneumencephalography, transcallosal puncture, sympathectomy, carotidal ligature, adrenectomy, transplantation of endocrinous tissue, and peripheral operations in reflex epilepsy, that have still been advocated as therapeutic measures. Apart from a few special situations, all of these methods have been dismissed by the authors. Krause and Schum aimed at the epileptogenic focus and let no doubt that excision of the "primary convulsing center" is the only effective therapy. The location of the epileptogenic area was achieved by electrical stimulation of the exposed motor cortex. At about the same time as Krause, Otfried Foerster of Breslau focussed on the semiology of seizures and its localizing significance [8]. Based on the cortical map of O. Vogt, his case reports include precise conclusions with respect to the cortical field from which the seizures originate. An excellent overview has been provided by Wolf [25].

Epilepsy surgery was essentially stimulated after availability of the EEG, and the developmental impetus of both shifted from Europe to North America, especially to Montreal. By working with Foerster, Wilder Penfield became familiar with the use of electrical stimulation to map motor and sensory areas of the human cortex. However, Penfield went beyond Foerster by mapping other areas of the cortex that subserve speach, hearing, vision and, perhaps most crucial of all, memory function. In 1939 he started to surgically approach the anterior temporal lobe [16]. Penfield's coworker Herbert Jasper stressed the importance of special distribution of EEG-findings to localize the epileptic focus [17].

Corpus callosum section for treatment of epilepsy was first introduced by van Wagenen and Herren when, in 1940, they reported on 10 patients [23]. The idea underlying this procedure was that consciousness should not be lost if the seizure could be confined to one hemisphere. This hypothesis was based on the observation that generalized convulsions become less common when the corpus callosum has been destroyed by tumor or hemorrhage.

Even though McKenzie in Toronto was the first to report on hemispherectomy for control of seizures in 1938, it was after Krynow's report in 1950 [12] that hemispherectomy in infantile hemiplegia associated with seizures became widely used. The early results following hemispherectomy were so favorable that many centers throughout the world became interested in this procedure.

The classical epilepsy surgical program had thus been completed.

Epidemiology

Epilepsy is characterized by recurrent epileptic seizures. The prevalence of epilepsy accounts for 0.7% of the population. Incidence of epilepsy has been reported to range around 50/100.000 of the population per year. Despite optimal treatment, epilepsy is medically resistant in approximately 20% of cases. For at least 10% of these medically resistant patients, a focal seizure origin is postulated [7].

Surgical interventions represent a reasonable alternative to long-term antiepileptic drug therapy in those patients destined to achieve incomplete control of seizures. It seems obvious to assume that the earlier in the course of the illness a surgical intervention can be implemented, the more likely an individual can be restored to a useful and normal life. In consequence, the surgical treatment of epilepsies in childhood has gained increasing interest.

Presurgical Assessment of the Epileptogenic Zone

Having emphasized the need for considering intractable seizure patients as candidates for epilepsy surgery, clear criteria must be met. The presurgical work-up of candidates represents the first and most important phase of the epilepsy surgical program.

The focus of the presurgical evaluation is the accurate definition of the epileptogenic zone. According to Lueders and Awad [13] the following, closely related concepts should be defined and their mutual relationships clarified: *Irritative zone, pacemaker-zone, epileptogenic lesion, ictal symptomatogenic zone,* and *functional deficit zone* (Fig. 1).

The *irritative zone* is defined as the region of the cortex that generates interictal epileptiform discharges in the EEG. A major limitation of the concept of

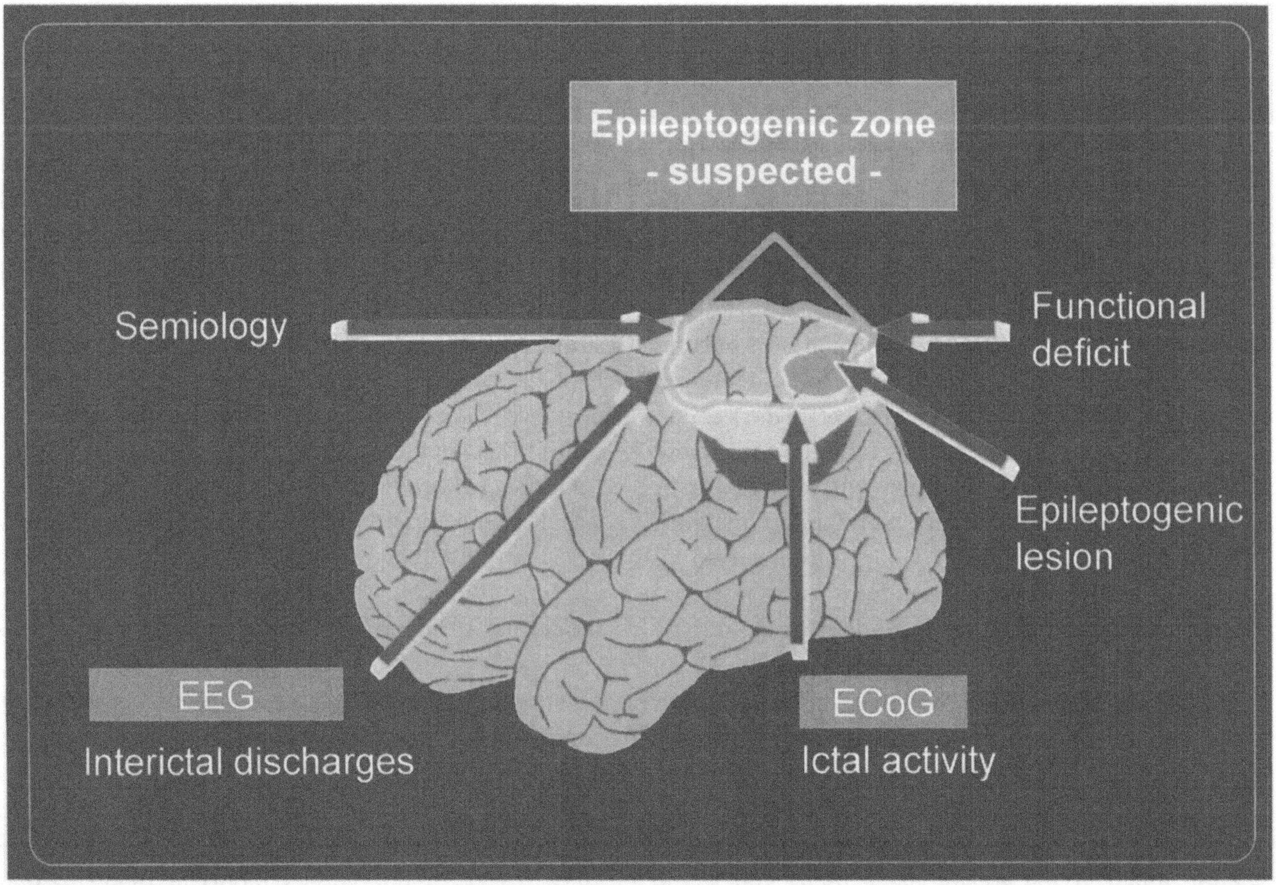

Fig. 1. Definition of the epileptogenic area (modified according to Lüders [8]

the irritative zone is that it is dependent on the definition of interictal epileptiform discharge, which is highly subjective when analyzed by different electroencephalographers. Another problem relates to the recording method used (non-invasive versus invasive recordings).

The *epileptogenic zone* represents the region of the cortex that can generate epileptic seizures. By definition total removal or disconnection of the epileptogenic zone is necessary and sufficient to achieve seizure relief.

The *pacemaker-zone* is defined as the region of the cortex from which the clinical seizures originate. Methods used to define the pacemaker-zone all have significant limitations. One of the main problems of electroencephalographic techniques is that non-invasive EEG is too insensitive to pick up the usually very limited area of cortex that represents the pacemaker-zone, and that invasive EEG-techniques will only define this area if they are exactly placed over the brain tissue from where seizures originate.

The *epileptogenic lesion* represents a brain lesion that is causative of the seizure disorder. The epileptogenic lesion is usually defined by neuroimaging. However, the spacial relationship between the epileptogenic lesion and the pacemaker-zone may be quite variable. Not infrequently, the two zones are not overlapping but immediately adjacent.

The *ictal symptomatogenic zone* is the region of cortex that generates the initial seizure symptomatology. For this reason the initial symptomatology of seizure is particularly important to define the epileptogenic zone, whereas later symptomatology tends to have only lateralizing value. However, the assumption that initial symptomatology of a seizure is a good index of the pacemaker-zone is certainly not correct in the majority of cases.

The *functional deficit zone* is defined as a region of cortex that in the interictal period is functioning abnormally as determined by neurological examination, neuropsychological testing, or functional neuroimaging. The location and extent of the functional deficit zone will depend on the destructive effect of the underlying structural lesion, the local and remote disturbance of brain function produced by the irritative zone, and possibly the long-lasting after-effects of frequent seizures that may persist into the so called interictal period.

In all, despite availability of sophisticated techniques, the definition of the epileptogenic zone remains hypothetical. It is clear that the success of any surgery with respect to risk and benefit will depend on how exactly the epileptogenic zone has been identified. This leads to the second phase of the epilepsy surgical program, the surgical intervention.

Principles of Surgical Treatment

Surgical interventions with a curative aim include temporal and extratemporal resections, and hemispherectomy. Recently, radiosurgery has been introduced aiming at complete seizure relief. On the other hand, callosotomy, multiple subpial transections and vagal nerve stimulation are summarized as palliative procedures aiming at significant improvement of the seizure status. According to large series, approximately 2/3 of all surgical procedures refer to the temporal lobe. Extratemporal resections account for about 20% of surgical interventions, whereas the remaining procedures refer to hemispherectomy, callosotomy, multiple subpial transections, vagal nerve stimulation, and radiosurgery [7].

Temporal Resections

Several approaches to the temporal lobe are available: Anterior temporal lobectomy (standard or key-hole) with or without hippocampectomy, extended lesionectomy with or without hippocampectomy and selective amygdalohippocampectomy. Standard anterior temporal lobectomy includes the removal of the anterior 4 to 5 cm of the temporal lobe followed by removal of the amygdala, the hippocampus and the parahippocampal gyrus. Although classical anterior temporal lobectomy is still widely used, there is a tendency to smaller resection types. Progress in the imaging and functional diagnostics has progressively allowed for a better localization of ictogenic areas and this enables more taylored resections. The key-hole approach has been designed to restrict removal of the temporal neocortex to a minimum while focussing on resection of mesiotemporal structures. Extended lesionectomy means complete removal of a lesion which may be combined with amygdalohippocampectomy. Selective amygdalohippocampectomy aims at removal of the mesiotemporal structures which are considered to be critical in the epileptogenesis while completely sparing the temporal neocortex [20, 27].

Since the introduction of selective amygdalohippocampectomy by Niemeyer [15] using the transcortical

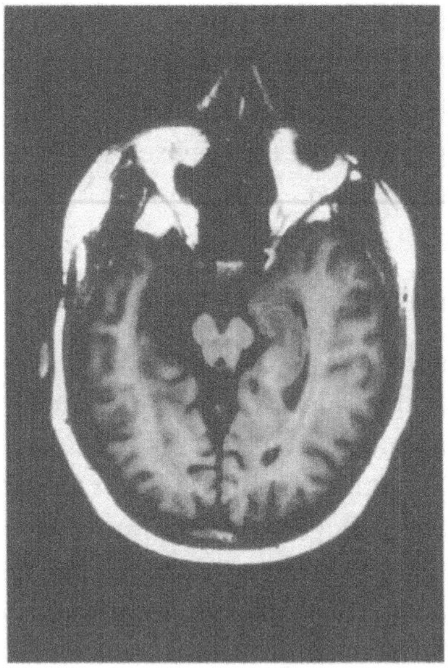

Fig. 2. Postoperative MRI after right-sided transsylvian selective amygdalohippocampectomy

approach, several modifications have been published: the transsulcal, the subtemporal and the transsylvian routes. The transcortical and transsulcal routes are technically more feasible, but they produce anavoidable damage to the lateral temporal neocortex. The subtemporal approach requires considerable retraction of the temporal lobe with potential injury to the vein of Labbé and the inferior temporal gyrus. The transsylvian approach as proposed by Yasargil (24, Fig. 2) seems to be the most adequate technique, but needs dissection of the Sylvian fissure with the risk of vascular complications. Other disadvantages of the transsylvian route include the limited space for dissection and difficulties in removal of posterior compartments.

Extratemporal Resections

The relatively low rate of extratemporal resections compared to procedures in the temporal lobe reflects not only differences in the epileptogenic potential of different brain areas. It also reflects the difficulty in managing extratemporal epilepsies. The most common problems encountered in evaluating patients with extratemporal seizure foci for surgery include poor EEG-localization of interictal spikes and of seizure onset, the presence of widespread, often ill-defined epileptogenic area, and the extension of the proposed area of resection into brain areas of high functionality. These characteristics of extratemporal epileptogenic foci are major obstacles to their successful surgical treatment [28].

Even in lesional cases, assessment of extratemporal epilepsies frequently requires intracranial recording of interictal activity and ictal events. The extent of the resection can be determined by either extraoperative localization techniques or by intraoperative electrocorticography. In our experience, intraoperative electrocorticography is sufficient to delineate the boundaries of the resection in patients in whom a clear hypothesis as to the location of the epileptogenic zone has been obtained from non-invasive recordings and MRI-studies. In cases of an ill-defined epileptogenic area, extraoperative invasive recordings using strip and grid electrodes should be preferred [28].

In addition to recording interictal and ictal activity, extraoperative functional mapping can be performed by stimulating contacts of implanted electrodes and by recording evoked potentials. By using convergent information from non-invasive and invasive recordings, including functional testing, maps may be constructed delineating the area of resection in relation to structural lesions and brain areas of high functionality (Fig. 3). Thus, the extent of the resection can be defined according to EEG-data and information regarding structural and functional localization, as proposed by Davies and Weeks [5]. Alternatively, functional mapping can also be performed intraoperatively in awake patients by using local anesthesia. We have not used this approach in our patients.

Callosotomy

The corpus callosum is the most important commissure of the human brain and connects homotopic fields of the neocortex, thus representing a neencephalic part of the telencephalon. Although the nature of synaptic organization is not fully understood, electrical stimulation of callosal axons leads to excitatory and inhibitory responses. Stimulated by the experimental literature which suggests an important role of the corpus callosum in seizure spread, callosotomy has gained interest in the treatment of medically intractable seizures not amenable to resective surgery. During the last decades, this procedure has undergone continuous change, and the numbers of structures divided have steadily decreased. At the present time, anterior, posterior and total corpus callosum sections are the procedures most widely practised, and the anterior

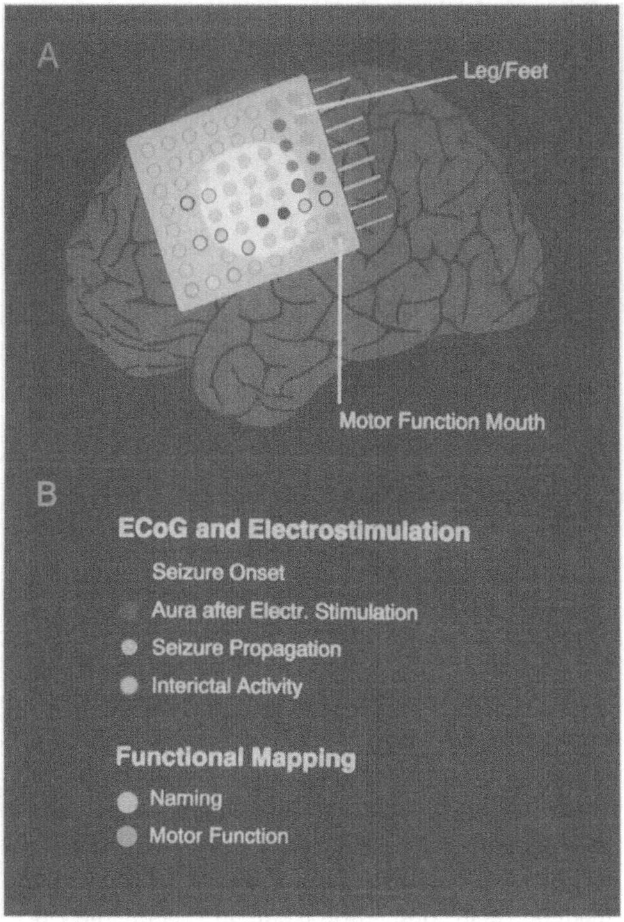

Fig. 3. Recording of the zone of seizure onset and functional topographic mapping in a patient with extratemporal epilepsy

commissure, fornix and massa intermedia are spared (29, Fig. 4).

Hemispherectomy

Hemispherectomy has proven to be a very valuable procedure in the management of epilepsies due to unilateral hemispheric disease such as hemiatrophy or hemimegalencephaly. Avoiding superficial cerebral hemosiderosis often seen following the classical anatomical hemispherectomy while providing the patients with the best seizure control, has been the objective of different hemispherectomy techniques described so far [22].

In the Oxford modification [1] the resection cavity is reduced by creating a large extradural space and by separating the subdural cavity from the ventricular system. Hemidecortication is carried out removing cortex and leaving white matter as well as the deep grey matter, thus leaving significant brain volume. Rasmussen [19] proposed a subtotal anatomical but complete physiological hemispherectomy that he termed functional hemispherectomy. This Montreal modification which today is most frequently used includes removal of the temporal and parietal lobes, whereas the frontal and occipital lobes are preserved but disconnected. Leaving these disconnected portions of the hemisphere within the cranial cavity, no large space is left behind.

Although the methods are different, these techniques should have exactly the same result toward seizure control for a given indication, since the physiological result is identical to the anatomical hemispherectomy. The techniques differ in a way that they aim at preventing superficial cerebral hemosiderosis. Recently, a new technique has been described which aims at disconnecting the whole hemisphere using a transsylvian-transventricular approach, thus avoiding brain resection [21]. It has been shown that this technique provides essential advantages over conventional methods by significantly shortening the operation time and reducing the blood loss (Fig. 5).

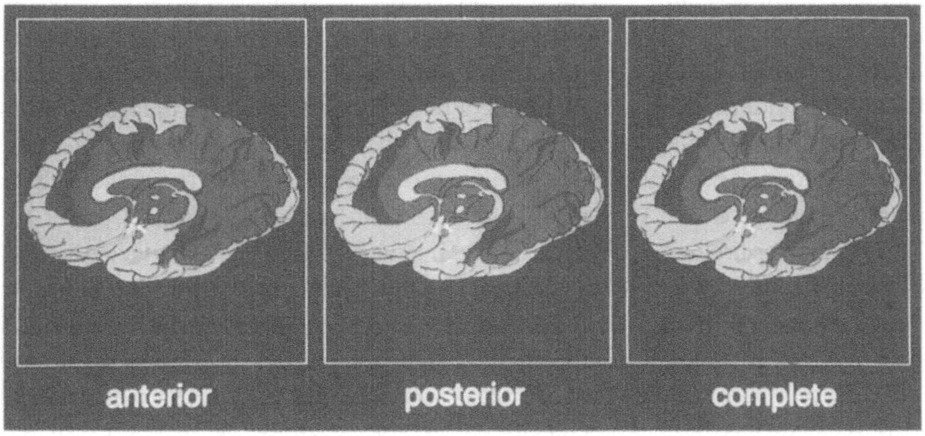

Fig. 4. Schematic representation of variants of corpus callosum section

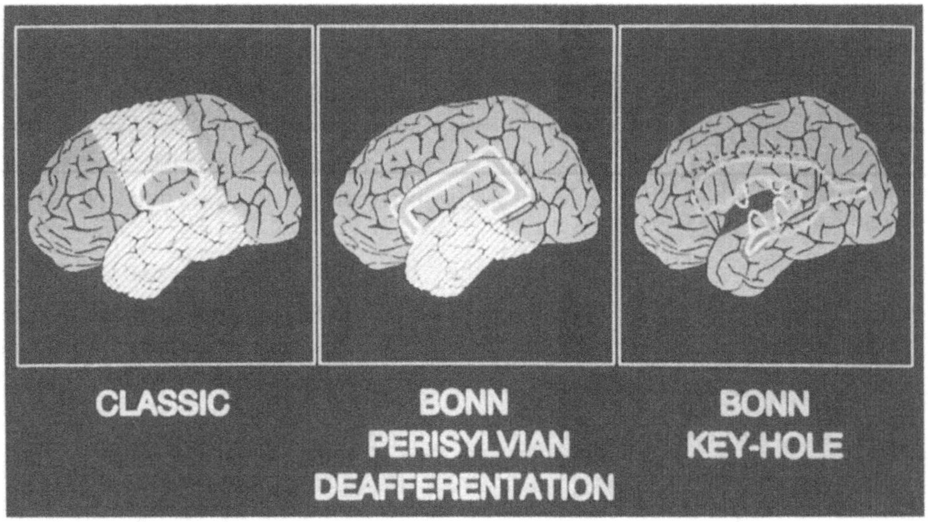

Fig. 5. Schematic representation of variants of functional hemispherectomy

Alternative Surgical Techniques

Alternative surgical techniques include deep brain stimulation, vagal nerve stimulation, stereotactic amygdalotomy and multiple subpial transections.

The use of chronic cerebellar stimulation as a therapy for intractable seizures is based on studies with animal models. In these models it has been shown that stimulation of vermis and intermediate cortex is more efficacious than stimulation of the lateral hemisphere. Moreover, chronic cerebellar stimulation is more effective in models of generalized or focal epilepsies of the limbic system and less effective in models of focal epilepsies of the sensory-motor cortex. Human studies have shown that chronic cerebellar stimulation may be offered to patients with intractable seizures originating from bilateral or extratemporal foci. Although nonblinded clinical reports are encouraging, double-blind studies showed no benefit [26].

Classical experiments by Dempsey and Morrison [6] demonstrated that the stimulation of the midline thalamus in cats influence cortical EEG. A possible relation of thalamic electrical activity to certain types of epilepsy has been the subject of experimentation and speculation for decades. Based on promising preliminary results, a group at Johns Hopkins in Baltimore tested electrostimulation of the centromedian nucleus of thalamus in a double-blind protocol. Improvement was not significant.

In animal experiments, the vagus nerve has been known for many years to influence the EEG. At low intensities and frequencies the stimulation excites large fibres and this leads to EEG synchronization. At higher stimulation intensities and frequencies the result is EEG desynchronization. Vagal nerve stimulation in patients with intractable epilepsy was initiated at the end of 1988 [18]. It has been shown that chronic intermediate vagal stimulation is safe in general and efficacious in reducing seizure frequency in a significant number of patients. There is a need for better means of identifying the best clinical candidates and the most effective stimulation parameters.

Stereotactic amygdalotomy was first introduced as a treatment for behaviour disorders. Improvement in seizures was observed additionally in parallel to improvement in behaviour. Subsequently, several groups reported series of amygdalotomies for epilepsy. Introduction of the stereotactic EEG recording method by Bancaud and Talairach [3] made it possible to record from depth wires in the vicinity of the amygdala. In consequence a combination of stereotactic recording and lesioning has been advocated for the treatment of seizures. Seizures originating from one or both amygdalae are rare but such patients are the most likely to benefit from stereotactic amygdalotomy [2].

Resection of cerebral tissue has the inevitable consequence that all functions subserved by that tissue are lost. Therefore removal of an epileptogenic zone that happens to lie in speach cortex or primary motor and sensory areas is not a real option for patients with medically intractable seizures. A new surgical approach referred to as multiple subpial transections

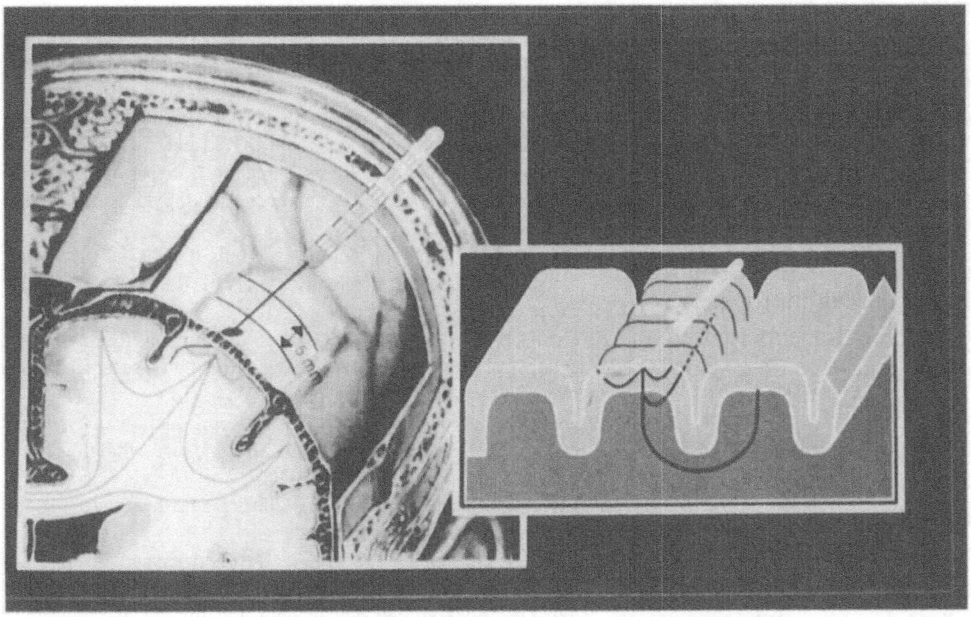

Fig. 6. Schematic representation of multiple subpial transections. Cortical incisions are made in 5 mm-intervals (according to 14)

(MST) has been developed by Morrell and colleagues in this situation (14, Fig. 6). The rationale behind the invention of this approach was evidence from Morell's laboratory indicating that there was a critical mass of side-to-side connectivity that was necessary for the generation of an epileptic spike. Moreover, it has been shown that the main functional attributes of cerebral cortical tissue depends upon vertically oriented cortical colums. Morell reasoned that a surgical method, which disrupted horizontal and tangential fibres but did not interfer with the basic columna organisation of the axons feeding into or out of the cortical columns, might eliminate the capacity for epileptogenic discharge without impairing the principal physiological action of cerebral cortex. The technique involves the selective interruption of the short horizontal, intracortical fibres at 5 mm intervals along those gyri excipiting electrocorticographically recorded epileptiform activity. Critical features of the procedure are the strict sparing of vertically oriented incoming and outgoing neural elements, and minimal trauma to the cortical blood supply. Indeed, it has been shown that MST leaves normal function intact and only subtile and not disabling deficits may remain in some cases. Thus, MST permits an extention of surgical treatment to brain regions so far considered inoperable. Although improvement in seizure frequency is observed in a significant number of patients, the operation usually is not curative.

Results

The evaluation of postoperative results and patients' care after surgery forms the third phase of the epilepsy surgical program. The following aspects are of particular importance: Seizure situation, operative complications, and neuropsychological performance.

Epileptological results of different surgical procedures vary within a large range and mainly depend on criteria used for selection of surgical candidates. In general, the prognosis for seizure control is more favorable when seizures are related to a well circumscribed structural lesion such as Ammon's horn sclerosis, tumors or non-tumorous lesions. Complete removal of those lesions provides the best basis for seizure control. Moreover, resection of the zone of seizure origin and the zone of maximal interictal spiking has been shown to improve seizure prognosis [7].

According to large series, most favorable epileptological results have been observed in temporal resections including selective amygdalohippocampectomy as well as in hemispherectomy. With these procedures, 70–80% of patients become completely seizure-free, and 10–20% are significantly improved. Thus, about 90% of the patients can be expected to noticeably benefit from surgery. Extratemporal resections are generally not as successful as temporal lobe resections. Complete seizure control is observed in 60–70%, and 70–80% of the patients will noticeably benefit from surgery. With palliative procedures such as callosotomy, multiple subpial transections, and vagal nerve stimulation, complete seizure control is only occasionally observed. However, approximately half of the patients significantly improve after surgery [7].

Obviously, postoperative neurological complications depend on the type of the procedure and mainly refer to hemiparesis, hemianopsia, oculomotor nerve paresis, and speach disturbances. In experienced hands, such complications range between 2–4%, while mortality is below 1%. Callosotomy may be followed by an acute disconnection syndrome, which is largely reversible in most cases, lasting for days to weeks and which is related to the extent of section. The possibility of a disabling split-brain-syndrome and deficit reinstatement after complete callosotomy highlights the necessity to evaluate callosotomy candidates for structural lesions and abnormalities of functional organisation [4].

The postoperative neuropsychological situation is a matter of major concern, particularly after extensive resections of limbic structures on the dominant side, e.g. extensive left-sided hippocampectomies. Although we do not face significant neurological deterioration in the great majority of our patients, such complications may be disabling for some patients and interfere with daily life activities. Therefore, great attempts are undertaken by epileptologists and neuropsychologists to preoperatively recognize patients, who are in danger of neuropsychological complications and accordingly to modify surgical strategies. Event-related potentials seem to be a promising tool in this context [7].

Conclusions

Epilepsy surgery has proven to be a highly effective treatment option for a minority of patients with epilepsy resistant to medical therapy. However, the epilepsy surgical program is very complex, since it not only requires an expensive technical equipment and interaction of several disciplines, but also the know-how of highly specialized personnel. Therefore, the epilepsy surgery program should be restricted to a few centers, where sufficient experience is available to manage even most difficult cases. Under these conditions, the cost-benefit-ratio can be expected to speak in favor of surgical treatment. Therefore, we should no longer hesitate to offer our epilepsy patients the chance of seizure control by a surgical procedure.

References

1. Adams CBT (1983) Hemispherectomy – a modification. J Neurol Neurosurg Psychiatry 46: 617–619
2. Andy OJ, Jurko MF, Hughes JR (1975) Amygdalotomy for bilateral temporal lobe seizures. South Med J 68: 743–748
3. Bancaud J, Talairach J, Bonis J, Schaub A, Szikla C, Morel G, Bordos-Ferrer M (1965) La stereoencephalopylie dans l'epilepsie. Masson, Paris
4. Behrens E, Schramm J, Zentner J, König R (1997) Surgical and neurological complications in a series of 708 epilepsy surgery procedures. Neurosurgery 41: 1–10
5. Davies KG, Weeks RD (1993) Cortical resections for intractable epilepsy of extratemporal origin: experience with seventeen cases over eleven years. Br J Neurosurg 7: 343–353
6. Dempsey EW, Morison RS (1942) Reproduction of rhythmically recurrent cortical potentials after localized thalamic stimulation. Am J Physiol 135: 293–300
7. Elger CE, Schramm J (1993) Chirurgische Epilepsietherapie. Radiologe 33: 165–171
8. Foerster O, Penfield W (1930) Der Narbenzug am und im Gehirn bei traumatischer Epilepsie in seiner Bedeutung für das Zustandekommen der Anfälle und für die therapeutische Bekämpfung derselben. Zschr Ges Neurol Psychiat 125: 475–572
9. Heikkinen ER, Heikkinen MI, Sotaniemi K (1992) Stereotactic radiotherapy instead of conventional Epilepsy surgery. Acta Neurochir 119: 159–160
10. Horsley V (1886) Brain-surgery. Br Med J 2: 670–674
11. Krause F (1911) Chirurgie des Gehirns und Rückenmarks nach eigenen Erfahrungen. Urban, Schwarzenberg Berlin
12. Krynauw RA (1950) Infantile hemiplegia treated by removing one cerebral hemisphere. J Neurol Neurosurg Psychiatry 13: 243–267
13. Lüders HO, Awad I (1992) Conceptual considerations. In: Lüders HO (ed) Epilepsy surgery. Raven Press, New York, pp 51–62
14. Morrell F, Whisler WW, Bleck TP (1989) Multiple subpial transection: a new approach to the surgical treatment of focal epilepsy. J Neurosurg 70: 231–239
15. Niemeyer P (1958) The transventricular amygdalohippocampectomy in temporal lobe epilepsy. In: Baldwin M, Bailey P (eds) Temporal lobe epilepsy. CC Thomas, Springfield, pp 461–482
16. Penfield W (1939) The epilepsies: with a note on radical therapy. N Engl J Med 221: 209–218
17. Penfield W, Jasper H (1954) Epilepsy and the functional anatomy of the human brain. Little, Brown Boston
18. Penry JK, Deen JC (1990) Prevention of intractable partial seizures by intermittent vagal stimulation in humans: preliminary results. Epilepsia 32: 40–43
19. Rasmussen T (1983) Hemispherectomy for seizures revisited. Can J Neurol Sci 10: 71–78
20. Spencer DD, Inserni J (1992) Temporal lobectomy. In: Lüders H (ed) Epilepsy surgery. Raven Press, New York, pp 533–546
21. Schramm J, Behrens E, Entzian W (1995) Hemispherical deafferentation: an alternative to Functional hemispherectomy. Neurosurgery 36: 509–516
22. Villemure JG (1992) Hemispherectomy techniques. In: Lüders HO (ed) Epilepsy surgery. Raven Press, New York, pp 569–578
23. Wagenen WP van, Herren RY (1940) Surgical division of commissural pathways in the corpus callosum, relation to spread of an epileptic attack. Arch Neurol Psychiatry 44: 740–759

24. Wieser HG, Yasargil MG (1982) Selective amygdalohippocampectomy as a surgical treatment of mediobasal limbic epilepsy. Surg Neurol 17: 445–457
25. Wolf P (1992) The history of surgical treatment of epilepsy in Europe. In: Lüders H (ed) Epilepsy surgery. Raven Press, New York, pp 9–18
26. Wright GD, McLellan DL, Brice JG (1984) A double-blind trial of chronic cerebellar stimulation in twelve patients with severe epilepsy. J Neurol Neurosurg Psychiatry 47: 769–774
27. Zentner J, Hufnagel A, Wolf HK, Ostertun B, Behrens E, Campos MG, Solymosi L, Elger CE, Wiestler OD, Schramm J (1995) Surgical treatment of temporal lobe epilepsy: Clinical, radiological and histopathological findings in 178 patients. J Neurol Neurosurg Psychiatry 58: 666–673
28. Zentner J, Hufnagel A, Ostertun B, Wolf HK, Behrens E, Campos MG, Solymosi L, Elger CE, Wiestler OD, Schramm J (1996) Surgical treatment of extratemporal epilepsy: Clinical, radiological and histopathological findings in 60 patients. Epilepsia 37: 1072–1080
29. Zentner J (1997) Surgical aspects of corpus callosum section. In: Tuxhorn I, Holthausen H, Boenigk H (eds) Paediatric epilepsy syndromes and their surgical Treatment. John Libbey, London, pp 830–839

Correspondence: Prof. Dr. J. Zentner, Univ. Klinikum Freiburg, Abt. Allg. Neurochirurgie im Neurozentrum, Breisacher Straße 64, 79106 Freiburg I. BR., Germany.

Acta Neurochir (2002) [Suppl] 84: 37–47

Gamma Knife Surgery, a Neuromodulation Therapy in Epilepsy Surgery!

J. Régis[1,2], F. Bartolomei[2,3], M. Hayashi[1,4], and P. Chauvel[2,3]

[1] Stereotactic and Functional Neurosurgery Department, Timone Hospital, Marseilles France
[2] Neurophysiology/Neuropsychology INSERM 9926, Timone Hospital, Marseilles France
[3] Neurophysiology Department, Timone Hospital, Marseilles France
[4] Neurosurgery Department Tokyo Women's Medical University, Tokyo, Japan

Summary

Introduction. The more classical approach for Epilepsy surgery is the removal of the epileptogenic zone (ZE). We present a critical review of information in favor of a possible non-destructive effect of radiosurgery in epilepsy surgery.

Material. Clinical material of patients with epilepsies related to a lesion in highly functional areas subjected to radiosurgery with relief of the seizures and no functional worsening is available. We applied direct treatment of the EZ with good efficacy in the absence of destructive aspects on the MR and no functional deterioration (eg hypothalamic hamartomas). Experimental studies have shown biochemical differential effect of radiosurgery on the striatum, glial cell elimination, stem cell migration toward the target area, sprouting,... Plasticity phenomenon are induced by radiosurgery when using non necrotizing dosemetry.

Discussion. There is clinical and experimental evidence of Gamma Knife capability to induce modulation in the neural system. Detailed mechanism of this modulation and dosemetric parameters enabling to induce such plasticity with no necrosis are still unknown. Subpial transection turning out actually to be quite disappointing, there is a specific rationale to test radiosurgery capability to treat EZ cortex while preserving the underlying function of this cortex when the functional risk for cortectomy is too high.

Keywords: Epilepsy; neuromodulation; radiosurgery; entorhinal area.

Introduction

Considerable interest has been generated over the past decade as regards the surgical treatment of medically intractable epilepsy. Advances in our understanding of seizure disorders and in neuroimaging, and wider appreciation by both physicians and the public of what may be accomplished by surgery have led to considerable growth in the number and activity of comprehensive epilepsy programs around the world.

In parallel with the development of such sophisticated diagnostic tools as long-term video-EEG monitoring, high resolution magnetic resonance imaging (MRI), and ictal single photon emission computed tomography (SPECT), there have also been major advances in therapeutic modalities. Within the operating room, refinement of the operating microscope, the introduction of interactive image guided surgery and the evolution of neuroanesthesia, to cite just a few examples, have made surgical address of the epileptogenic zone a routine and acceptably safe procedure.

The initial radiosurgical instrument developed by Lars LEKSELL around 1950 was dedicated to Functional Neurosurgery [30] and the first patients operated on were suffering from trigeminal neuralgia [31] and parkinsonism [33]. LEKSELL's team were subsequently able to perform thalamotomies for tremors or for intractable pain and capsulotomies for psychiatric disorders [32]. This clinical experience showed that Gamma Knife could induce precise and well-defined small-volume lesions. The absence of mortality, the very low morbidity, and the comfort of the patient are most pertinent factors for functional neurosurgery. Over a long period, due to absence of high-quality images, Gamma Knife Surgery was mainly used for treatment of AVMs and tumors. The availability of high-quality 3D imaging with MR (for precise targeting of normal structures) and evidence of some limitations regarding drug efficacy have now prompted a reappraisal of Gamma Knife surgery for functional disorders [33, 36]. Between 1955 and 1973, Talairach and colleagues treated 44 epileptic patients by stereotactic implantation of Yttrium 90 into the amygdala and the hippocampus [67]. Two patients in this series experienced hemiparesis due to anterior choroid artery occlusion. These technical difficulties, related to the use of the radioelement, led to subsequent abandonment of this approach, however, first clinical results were promising [67].

A few years later Steiner and Lindquist, analyzing their clinical experience with arteriovenous malformations (AVM), noted that epilepsy was frequently improved after GK surgery [22, 35, 65, 66]. Of 247 patients treated between 1970 and 1984 by GK surgery in Stockholm, 59 had seizures. Fifty-two of these patients (88%) observed disappearance of the latter. Frequently seizure cessation occurred several months before occlusion of the AVM, and in three cases in spite of failure to obtain occlusion [33]. Lindquist subsequently promoted the idea that GK was perhaps an interesting new approach for epilepsy surgery, although his first attempts to treat epileptic nonlesional patients were not encouraging [2, 33].

Disappearance of seizures after radiosurgical treatment of a lesion when the patient presented with seizures was reported by other teams [22, 70, 71]. A similar observation was made after brachytherapy [57], conformal radiotherapy [56], and conventional radiotherapy [56]. Barcia-Salorio reported in a short abstract the antiepileptic potential of ionizing radiation in an experimental cat model of epilepsy [7]. The same author, since 1985, has published in several proceedings interesting clinical results but till now no peer reviewed paper has been issued [6].

Materials

Gamma Knife Surgery of Mesial Temporal Lobe Epilepsy

Several reasons led us to propose the evaluation of Gamma Knife Surgery in this indication. Mesial temporal lobe epilepsy (MTLE) is a very common, well-characterized, and often drug-resistant form of partial epilepsy with good surgical prognosis [15, 72]. MTLE has a good outcome following limited temporal lobe resection [73, 74], and today there is agreement that MTLE can be diagnosed in most patients without invasive tests [17, 72]. Several classic surgical strategies have been developed, with resection more or less limited to the temporomesial structures and a range of different approaches. The anterior temporal lobectomy (ATL) described by D. Spencer [61] is certainly the most frequently practised approach. We consider that the transsylvian amygdalohippocampectomy proposed by Yasargil is an interesting model in that the final volume of the resection was quite small and within the range of Gamma Knife capability [74].

Although the risk of epilepsy surgery is low, surgical complications may occur, such as postoperative neurologic deficit due to unintended vascular compromise or other accidental damage [19, 42, 62]. Another argument for choosing this group of patients is the fact that in the event of unexpected failure or complication it is always possible to remove the target by microsurgical salvage resection. As there have been no reports of successful attempts at treating MTLE by GK, the optimum target definition and technical parameters (dose, volume etc.) had to be chosen and, together with strict selection of patients, were obviously of crucial importance to success.

In March 1993 the first patient with medically refractory mesial temporal lobe epilepsy was treated by Gamma Knife surgery in Marseilles [53]. Instead of a microsurgical procedure, an entorhinoamygdalohippocampectomy was performed with the Gamma Knife at low marginal dose (25 Gy). The patient has been seizure-free since the day of treatment without any clinical complication [53]. To determine the best technical parameters for treatment, the same procedure was repeated in three other MTLE patients with slight changes, namely progressive decreases in target volume and dose. The quality of results decreased in proportion to dose and volume. After follow-up of these four patients over a two-year period, however, the safety and efficacy of this method led to a more extensive study.

The indication of this noninvasive surgery requires the same preoperative criteria as microsurgical amygdalahippocampectomy, with perfect agreement of all the electroclinical, radiological and metabolic data. Patients with space-occupying lesions and/or severe psychiatric disorders were excluded from this protocol.

The anatomical target includes the amygdaloid complex (sparing the upper and mesial part), the head and anterior half of the body of the hippocampus, and the anterior part of the parahippocampal gyrus. As previously suggested by Wieser for the microsurgical alternative [74] and by some experimental data, the anterior part of the entorhinal area was included within the target volume [75].

In the present protocol the target is covered by two 18 mm collimators, with a dose of 20 to 25 Gy at the 50% marginal isodose line. The target volume is 6500 to 7000 mm^3. It is important to consider that, with this protocol, the results have been very reproducible and, until now, failures have rarely been observed.

After Gamma Knife surgery patients were subjected to regular medical examination and waking EEG. The outcome of seizure was measured according to Engel's classification [16]. As the effectiveness of the procedure is delayed in time, direct use of the Engel scale is not realistic, and we therefore use a modified Engel scale score. MRI scans were performed regularly after Gamma Knife surgery. The radiosurgical treatment was carried out with the agreement of the ethics committee: (Comité Consultatif de Protection des Personnes dans la Recherche Biomédicale, Marseilles I, 1994 and 1996).

Twenty five patients were treated according to this protocol, and the follow-up for the entire group was between 12 and 72 months [49]. The follow up was superior to 2 years for 16 patients. Thirteen of these 16 (81%) patients are seizure free. The median latency in seizure cessation occurrence was 10,5 months (range 6–21) apart from two patients who were immediatly seizure free. The median latency in aura cessation was 15,5 months (range 9–22).

Apart from the two patients who, as noted, were seizure-free since the day of treatment, patients experienced a gradual decrease in the frequency, intensity and duration of seizures. No depression syndrome was observed. For some patients, a delay in seizure cessation is a source of anxiety. In the majority of cases, clear early changes in the seizures provided patients with confidence in the eventual result. The median delay in the appearance of the MRI changes was 10,5 months (range 7–22). During the period of onset of these radiological changes three patients experienced headache associated in two cases with nausea and vomiting. These signs resolved immediately after prescription of low doses of steroids [48, 49, 55]. Visual field deficit was observed in three cases (2 homonymous superior quadrantanopia and one hemianopia) and was symptomatic only in the latter case.

The chronology of MRI changes was quite reproducible from one patient to another. MRI examinations showed only a slightly increased T2 signal inside the target volume at six months. A contrast enhancement ring subsequently appeared, corresponding exactly to the periphery of the target region (50% isodose line). Outside the target volume there was a larger area of homogeneously increased T2W signal, predominantly affecting the white-matter tracts of the temporal lobe [55]. Corticosteroid treatment was routinely initiated at this time (methylprednisolone, 0.5 mg/kg/day) and gradually discontinued, depending on the MRI evolution.

The mechanism of action is not clear. The sudden onset of CT and MR changes after the treatment of large lesions such as AVM with 20 to 25 Gy in peripheral [65, 66] or small volumes of normal brain with very high doses ranging from 100 to 300 Gy [28, 34, 64, 77] has been well described. The structural significance of these aspects, called "radionecrosis" or "radioinduced edema", remains unclear. In some patients late MR control, after the disappearance of high T2 signal and contrast enhancement, demonstrated that the targeted structures were not destroyed. A series of arguments (see [50]) advocated that these images were not the unequivocal sign of radionecrosis, and the term "radioinduced MR changes" is preferable.

Efficacy appears to be comparable to that of microsurgical resection. The results of classic surgery for epilepsy show that nearly 75% of patients with temporal lobe epilepsy become seizure-free after surgery [16, 58, 62, 63]. Definite conclusions about Gamma Knife efficacy cannot be drawn due to the short-term follow-up, but our preliminary results of Gamma Knife "amygdalohippocampectomy" suggest that this method is as effective as the microsurgical approach. Secondary failures are, of course, still possible and a follow up longer than two years is probably necessary for a serious evaluation [14, 76].

Hypothalamic Hamartomas

Patients with Hypothalamic Hamartomas (HH) frequently present gelastic or more rarely dacrystic seizures [10, 25, 68]. Onset of epilepsy ranges from 1 day to 15 years in the literature (mean 2.8 years) [68]. Therefore, the evolution of the disease is considered as invariably unfavorable because of the occurrence of several types of seizures, the worsening of EEG features (progressively marked by generalized discharges) and the mental impairment. Brief gelastic seizures are generally the first to occur and are refractory to drug therapy. During evolution, gelastic seizures become more prolonged and complex and other types of intractable seizure generally occur including complex partial seizures with or without secondary generalization and tonic or tonicoclonic generalized seizures. Seizures with fall are described in 50% of cases in patients aged more than 15 years. In addition precocious puberty and progressive mental decline are commonly reported.

The responsibility of HH in the genesis of seizures was first suggested by the success in some patients of the resection of the HH itself [45–47]. The direct demonstration of the role of HH was obtained with data from stereo-EEG recordings. In patients with gelastic [40] or dacrystic [26] seizures, a low-voltage fast recruiting discharge was first recorded in the HH before the appearance of changes in other regions explored. Nevertheless microsurgical resection in this most critical area is related to a very high risk of occulomotor palsy, hemiparesis and visual field deficit, so that the majority of epilepsy surgeons have abandoned this approach. The onset of seizures in the HH and the high risk of resective surgery are good arguments for investigating the potential efficiency of Gamma Knife surgery in this indication. The two main difficulties are the close relation with the optic tract and chiasm, and the poor limitation of the upper part of the lesion, frequently undistinguishable from the surrounding hypothalamus.

A single case of successful treatment by Gamma Knife for seizure associated with an HH has been reported recently by Arita [4]. In order to evaluate the safety and efficacy of GKS in this unfrequent pathology we organized a multicenter retrospective study [44]. Among the 10 patients, sufficient follow up was available for 8 patients from 6 different Gamma Knife centers. It was superior to 12 months for the 8 patients with a median follow up of 28 months (mean range 12–71 months). All these patients had severe drug-resistant epilepsy including frequent gelastic and generalized tonic or tonicoclonic attacks. The median age was 18,5 (range 2–34) and 3 patients had precocious puberty. All the patients had sessile HH. The median marginal dose was 15,25 Gy (range 12–20). Two patients were treated twice (at 19 and 49 months) due to unsufficient efficacy. All the patients were improved. Four patients are seizure free (3 IA and 1 IB), one has rare nocturnal seizures (IID), one has some rare partial seizures (IIA) and no more generalized attacks and two are only improved with a reduction in frequency of seizures but persistance of some rare generalized seizures (IIIA). All these patients were suffering from a severe drugresistant epilepsy with gelastic seizures, other complex partial seizures and generalized seizures. No significant morbidity was reported in this series (a case of nondisabling poikilothermia). This study indicated a clear correlation between some dosemetry parameters and changes of seizure cessation, peculiarly a higher marginal dose. The marginal dose (or cumulate marginal dose) was superior to 17 Gy for all the patients in the successful group and inferior to 13 Gy for all the patients in the "improved" group. Behavior was clearly improved in two patients (with only improvement of their epilepsy). Complete coverage of the HH does not seem to be mandatory since in two patients from the successful group, the dosemetry spared a significant part of the lesion. This series was the very first to demonstrate that Gamma Knife Surgery can constitute a safe and effective treatment for epilepsy when related to HH.

Callosotomies

Four attempts at Gamma Knife callosotomy were performed in Graz [41]. Two patients were treated with large volumes (3.7 cc)/low dose (50 Gy maximum) using an 8 mm collimator six times. Due to the absence of a good short term effect, a second procedure was performed in one of these two patients (0.35 cc, with three 4 mm isocenters, 170 Gy maximum) and 10 months after seizure frequency was reduced (70%). Two patients, both suffering from Lennox Gastaut syndrome, were treated with a small volume (0.45 cc)/ high doses (150/160 Gy maximum) using a 4 mm collimatore four times. Two and three months after GK surgery contrast enhancement appeared. Between the 3rd and 18th month postradiosurgery, the frequency of generalized tonicoclonic and atonic seizures gradually decreased (60–80%).

Cavernous Angiomas

Cavernous angioma (CA) may cause hemorrhage and repetitive neurological deficits, but the symptom most frequently presented is epilepsy [38]. In one large recent series, 40% of patients with supratentorial CA presented with drug-resistant epilepsy [11]. The general consensus is that microsurgical resection of the lesion is the choice treatment in patients with intractable epilepsy. For patients with seizures of recent onset in whom correlation between symptoms and the location of the CA is good, resection of the lesion itself is the best method (lesionectomy) [24]. Epilepsy surgery strategies should be preferred for patients with a long history of chronic epilepsy in whom correlation of clinical and electroencephelographic findings is unclear. In these cases a multimodal approach, including invasive techniques if necessary, should be considered. The adoption or nonadoption of these criteria probably explains why the success rate for surgical excision of CA varies from 20% to 80% in the literature [1, 11, 13, 18, 78].

Some authors have reported a decrease in bleeding after Gamma Knife surgery [29] while others have reported no effect [27, 60, 69]. Except for the special case of severe rebleeding of non-microsurgically resectable CA in the brainstem [29], radiosurgery is therefore not recommended to prevent the risk of bleeding in the case of supratentorial CA [27]. Furthermore, in some studies the incidence of radiation-induced complications was particularly high after GK treatment of CA [3, 27]. This effect must be limited by the use of a lower dose than that usually applied to other vascular targets.

The efficacy of the Gamma Knife in the management of seizures associated with cavernous angioma (CA) has been analyzed in a retrospective multicenter study [46]. The final study population consisted of 49 patients, with a mean age of 36 years at the time of Gamma Knife treatment. All the patients presented with seizures that were resistant to one or more antiepileptic drugs, and the mean duration of epilepsy before Gamma Knife treatment was 7.5 years ($\pm$9.3). The mean dose at the marginal isodose was 19.17 $\pm$ 4.4 Gy. With a mean follow-up of 23.66 $\pm$ 13 months after treatment, 26 patients (53%) are seizure-free including 24 class IA (49%) and 2 patients with occasional auras (class IB, 4%). A highly significant decrease in the number of seizures was achieved in ten patients (class IIB).

In the seizure-free group the mean delay between Gamma Knife treatment and complete remission was four months (range: 0 to 9 months, median 6 months). Location in the temporal region was associated with poor outcome (12/14). If we consider the population with CA, as regards extratemporal cortical areas, results turn out to be considerably better with 69.5% of the patients seizure-free. The results observed in this study are comparable to those reported for lesionectomy in the recent literature. The most valuable prognostic factor for the outcome of Gamma Knife treatment is the location of the lesion. A probable explanation for this finding is that the relationship between the lesion and the epileptogenic zone is particularly direct in primary areas such as the central region, but in contrast, when a CA is located in the mesial temporal region, the organization of the epileptogenic network is probably more complex.

Seven patients presented with major reactional edema during the first year after Gamma Knife surgery. In two of these cases manifestations were severe (hemiparesis and speech impairment), but all the patients recovered fully during follow-up. The low rate of radiation-induced complications in our series supports the idea that safe radiosurgery can be achieved by using Gamma Knife surgery at the state of the art with low marginal doses (<20 Gy). Although bleeding is more common with subcortical and infratentorial lesions, this risk is never negligible [43]. If the objective is to control bleeding, conventional microsurgery is the choice method. To date we consider the GK to be an alternative to conventional microsurgery in the treatment of epileptogenic CA in patients with CA in high risk locations such as the left temporal neocortex or rolandic cortex when electroclinical data show clear correlations.

Low-Grade Tumors

Whang *et al.* treated a series of patients with small benign lesions with the sole aim of curing the associated epilepsy [71]. Between June 1990 and May 1995 the authors treated 31 patients with such lesions, reportedly surrounded by a limited perilesional epileptogenic area on the basis of scalp EEG and MRI. 52% (12/23) became seizure-free after a follow-up of more than one year, 13% without medication (three patients). The difficulty in this series is to distinguish between failure due to insufficient radiosurgery and failure due to insufficient preoperative electroclinical analysis of the real spread of the epileptogenic area. Schröttner reported a retrospective analysis of 26 patients with cerebral tumors associated with intractable epilepsy. All these patients were treated by GK surgery for epilepsy control (there were 65% low grade gliomas). Results seem to be poor with 54% of the patients in class I+II of Engel. The original contribution of the paper is the analysis of the influence (on seizure cessation) of volume of surrounding cortex receiving doses superior to 10 Gray. The authors found that patients with a larger coverage of the surrounding cortex had a greater chance of seizure cessation [59].

Discussion

Epileptic Zone (EZ) turn out to be, in the majority of the patients with drug resistant epilepsy, a network of remote brain structures. In each area in which an element of this network is located, this element is surrounded by other structures not involved in the epileptic process. These structures are frequently involved in important functional capabilities and their removal is not necessary for surgical cure. "En Bloc" removal of the cortex including the epileptic network is the usual way to cure these patients by microsurgery. This large removal is not possible when highly functional areas are part of this "volume" and in other patients the cortectomy is not highly disabling but induce objective deterioration of elaborated cognitive processes!

Present Standards for Surgical Outcomes

For correct exploration of the role that new treatment may play in the management of any disease process, it is essential to establish first the standards or reasonable expectations of current conventional treatment. In as heterogeneous a field as intractable epilepsy, this requires consideration of a number of the most common epilepsy syndromes, each with its own management approach and degree of success. As a part of the Second Palm Desert International Conference on the Surgical Treatment of the Epilepsies held in 1992, Engel surveyed 100 epilepsy surgery centers who had treated 6,009 patients in the interval 1986–1990. The compiled results were grouped by surgical procedure and assessed seizure outcome. Anterior temporal lobectomy, performed in 3,579 patients, achieved a seizure-free outcome in 67.9%, an improved outcome in 24.0%, and no improvement in 8.1%. Selective amygdalo-hippocampectomy in 413 patients achieved seizure-free outcome in 68.8%, improvement in 22.3%, and no improvement in 9.0%. Lesionectomy in 293 patients rendered 66.6% seizure-free and 21.5% improved. Extratemporal resection rendered 45.1% of 805 patients seizure-free and improved 35.2%. Multilobar resection in 166 patients resulted in 45.2% seizure-free and 35.5% improved; hemispherectomy in 190 patients rendered 67.4% seizure-free and 21.1% improved. Corpus callosum section, generally recognized as a palliative procedure, achieved seizure-free outcome in only 7.6% of 563 patients, but 60.9% were improved [16].

The morbidity and mortality accompanying such surgeries must also be recognized. A meta-analysis compiled by Pilcher tabulated complications with many of the same procedures [42]. Reviewing anterior temporal lobectomy, the most common procedure of Engel's survey, he noted mortality of less than 1%, transient hemiparesis in 4%, permanent hemiparesis in 2%, mild visual field defects in more than 50%, severe field defects in 2–4%, infection in less than 0.5%. Transient anomia was found in more than 20%, but permanent language difficulty occurred in only 1–3%. Other epilepsy surgeries had more variable morbidities, depending on the region and extent of cortex involved [42]. In general, the surgical complications for epilepsy surgery have been reduced to very low but not negligible levels.

Strengths of the Microsurgical Approach

To achieve the level of success enjoyed today, the above surgical interventions took advantage of a number of opportunities provided by craniotomy. Exposure of the cortical surface itself enables utilization of intraoperative diagnostic techniques, most notably electrocorticography, that may guide resection. In a same context, cortical exposure allows intraoperative mapping of critical normal functions that must be preserved through such techniques as electrical stimulation and evoked potential recording.

Secondly, open techniques integrated with the magnification and illumination provided by today's operating microscopes enjoy outstanding visualization of the surgical field. This allows not only completeness of ablation, for example assurance of complete division of all intended callosal fibers for callosotomy, but also excellent protection of crucial but perhaps immediately adjacent structures that must be preserved. The latter may include the optic tract in medial temporal resection, the hippocampus in lateral temporal resection, language areas in temporal or frontal neocortical resection, and the fornices in callosotomy.

Thirdly, with the possible exception of the original hemispherectomy procedure, surgical resections are not limited regarding volumetric extent. In the more challenging cases of seizures associated with multilobar disease, surgical intervention in concert with functional localization may proceed unimpeded by physical dimension. Lastly, the benefits derived from surgical resection are generally obtained immediately.

Limitations of Surgery

There are clear limitations in all that can be accomplished by microsurgical intervention. The morbidities and mortality alluded to earlier are not inconsequential, particularly for what is usually an elective procedure. Related to this is the problem posed by pathologic processes in certain locations which render surgery a riskier undertaking. Resections in the hypothalamus, in portions of the insula and in the optic radiations, for examples, may entail substantially greater morbidity than that associated with other, more common interventions. For temporal lobe cortectomies, mortality related to microsurgical cortectomy or general anesthesia has decreased dramatically over recent decades but there is still a mortality of approximately 1% with open craniotomy [42]. In epileptic patients subjected to temporal lobe microsurgery in the retrospective comparative study of Guldov *et al.*, 23% had neurological deficits [19]. Half of these deficits in the surgically treated group interfered with function [19, 20]. The postoperative neurological status after temporal lobectomy was recently reviewed [62]. Transient hemiparesis was reported in 5% of patients. A superior homonymous quadrantanopsia was observed after temporal lobectomy in 50% of patients and was symptomatic in 8%. Transient aphasia could occur after dominant temporal lobectomy and was persistent in 3%. A disabling memory deficit was observed in 1% to 4% of patients.

Potential Advantages of Gamma Knife Treatment

Decreased Morbidity. No mortality and no major side-effect or morbidity has been observed in the Marseille mesial temporal lobe series [49]. Three patients experienced slight transient headache around the ninth month, which disappeared immediately after introduction of corticosteroid treatment. Neurological examination, including visual field, remained normal except in one patient with a superior homonymous quadrantanopia defect. No toxicity due to corticosteroid treatment was observed. In the group of 49 patients with cavernous angiomas and epilepsy described earlier, side-effects were limited to transient reactive edema in 7 patients [8].

Reasonably low and acceptable morbidity has characterized the Gamma Knife epilepsy experience to date, and this can be expected to decrease as appropriate indications and dose prescriptions become established.

Accessibity of Deep Sites. Related to the low morbidity associated with radiosurgical treatment is the ability to address lesions and epileptogenic regions that might be less easily approached microsurgically. The experience with hypothalamic hamartomas illustrates this, with the only morbidity observed in a group of ten patients being that of a single instance of non-disabling poikilothermia.

Potentially Non-Ablative Efficacy. Clinical experience with Gamma Knife in some epileptic lesions strongly suggests that the mechanisms of postradiosurgery epilepsy amelioration could constitute an actual antiepileptic effect. Indeed, epilepsy improvement was regularly observed despite the application of nonnecrotizing doses [5, 7, 44, 47, 48, 50, 51]. This is one of the most exciting aspects of the treatment, because it is then possible to treat epilepsy while sparing normal brain tissue and function.

Experimental data in this area are limited. Barcia-Salorio and colleagues used low-dose irradiation in a cobalt-induced epileptic cat model [7]. Within one month after irradiation with a total dose of 10 Gy, all EEG recordings returned to normal, while a control group maintained epileptic discharges. To better understand the dose response relationship between radiation and seizures, Mori and colleagues utilized a rat kainic acid model of chronic hippocampal epilepsy [39]. With randomization between control, 20, 40, 60, or 100 Gy, the study demonstrated increased response with higher doses and beneficial effect without tissue injury.

Chalifoux and Elisevich theorized that irradiation inhibited the protein synthesis necessary for the maintenance of spontaneous bursting [12]. A biochemical differential effect on the excitatory amino-acid system and the inhibitory GABA system has been suggested [51]. The biochemical differential effects obtained by radiosurgery suggest a potentially new way of using the Gamma Knife for the treatment of functional disorders with more selective action on the neuronal network.

In our series of MTLE morphological changes were for the majority reversible [21]. Mass effect disappeared completely at 22 months. Enhanced lesion decreased in size and some lesions disappeared (average 50.5 months) or reduce to a very small area. The others which have not yet disappeared are those with the shorter follow-up (average 32 months). This result infers absence of real tissue necrosis. Even in the cases with long-term residual MR lesion, the volume of this image is too small to explain the efficacy of GKS in curing epilepsy by a necrotizing effect of the target [21]. When such a residual small area in the center of the target remain enhanced by the gadolinium it is roughly corresponding to the 80% isodose line (40 Gy).

Limitations of Gamma Knife

Delayed Response. The clinical experience with Gamma Knife treatment and epilepsy has shown, with occasional exceptions, a latency of response of between 8 and 15 months. For a chronic disorder whose duration is almost always measured in terms of many years, such a delay in response may be more psychologically difficult than rationally problematic.

Volume Constraints. This is perhaps the main limit of GK. For the Marseille radiosurgical program we considered the target volume now used for mesial temporal lobe epilepsy (7 cc) as being a prudent volumetric limit. The seizure disorders whose anatomic and physiological substrate exceeds this or a similar threshold are not appropriate candidates for Gamma Knife epilepsy treatment.

The presence of MRI changes, with mass effect during several months (leading to steroid treatment during this period), has always been considered by us as unsatisfactory. Although clinical tolerance is good avoidance of these acute tissular changes should constitute an improvement. In a first period we decided to follow the same protocol in order to demonstrate, in a homogeneous series of patients, the safety efficacy of this protocol in cases with MTLE, as observed in the first patients. This series is now published [48] and confirms safety efficacy at short-middle term follow-up (minimum follow up 2 years). The analysis of our material and of some cases treated unsuccessfully throughout the world with different protocols has convinced us that the dose/volume effective window is very narrow and the risk of failure important when changing the dose or target.

We conclude that, in order to remain effective, it is probably important to respect the volume of the actual target. We recently treated some patients with the same dosemetry but with a lower marginal dose. First results seem to be promising but larger series and longer follow up are needed to evaluate the minimal doses threshold for reproducible efficacy on seizures. The second major problem for the definition of target volume is the appropriate anatomical delimitation of the epileptogenic zone (EZ). One should be very cautious in defining EZ without invasive recording (SEEG). The complexity of the epileptogenic zone in TLEs may be more important than it is usually thought. In particular, the epileptogenic zone may include complex interactions between mesial and neocortical structures [9, 23]. Targeting only the medial part of the temporal lobe by radio or micro surgery is probably a source of failure in these cases. The semiological difference is often subtle and when a doubt persists, we strongly promote the use of stereo-electroencephalography before GK to perfectly match the GK volume target and the EZ. This is particularly important with Gamma Knife because of the high selectivity of the procedure.

Conclusion

GKS constitutes a minimally invasive treatment for brain lesions. Safety, efficay, and comfort are promising as concerns application of this methodology in Epilepsy surgery. We first applied GKS for MTLE in 1993 and have gradually developed this concept and a dosemetric strategy. The field of application of GKS for epilepsy has spread to other epileptic syndromes such as hypothalamic hamartome or cavernous angiomas [44, 46]. However, the action mechanism, especially for MTLE, has not been elucidated [49]. The initial MR changes suggest necrosis [52, 55] but long-term follow-up provides us with opposite arguments. Why do patients experience seizure cessation before major morphological changes [52]? Surprisingly the patients operated on by Gamma Knife suffered less neuropsychological (mnesic) deterioration than those operated classically [49]. We also have experience of GKS in the treatment of epileptogenic lesions in highly functional areas with good antiepileptic effect and without functional worsening [45, 48]. The possibility of preserving the underlying function after treatment with GKS is potentially a great advantage over microsurgical cortectomies in functional areas [54]. Up to now, this remains more or less a speculation. Alternatively some experimental studies have been performed. We reported differential biochemical changes after GKS, while targeting rat striatum, with impairment of certain biochemical systems and apparent integrity of others [51]. Maesawa in a preliminary experimental study provided some confirmation of 2 of our observations in humans [37]. We have demonstrated that subnecrotic doses could cure or improve epilepsy without destruction of the tissue and without deterioration of underlying function [21]. The first successful case of epilepsy surgery (without space-occupying lesion) operated on by Gamma Knife (MTLE) was performed in Marseilles in 1993. Our first series is very encouraging but is limited by the low number of patients and the shortness of follow up. Longer follow-up and larger series are required to definitively evaluate what is still an experimental method but the evidence of a non destructive mechanism accounting for a part of the results on seizures is very appealing for future developments in Epilepsy Surgery.

Acknowledgment

We thank the "Assistance Publique des Hôpitaux de Marseille" which supported this work.

References

1. Acciari N, Giulioni M, Padovani R, Galssi E, Gaist G (1995) Surgical management of cerebral cavernous angiomas causing epilepsy. J Neurosurg Sci 39: 13–20
2. Alexander E, Lindquist C (1993) Special indications: radiosurgery for functional neurosurgery and epilepsy. In: Alexander E, III, Loeffler J, Lunsford L (ed) Stereotact radiosurg. Mc Graw-Hill, New York, pp 221–225
3. Amin-Hanjani S, Ogilvy CS, Candia GJ, Lyons S, Chapman PH (1998) Stereotactic Radiosurgery for cavernous malformations: Kjellberg's experience with proton beam therapy in 98 cases at Harvard cyclotron. Neurosurgery 42: 1229–1238
4. Arita K, Kurusi K, Iida K, Hanaya R, Akimitsu T, Hibino S, Pant B, Hamasaki M, Shinagawa S (1998) Subsidence of seizure induced by stereotactic radiation in a patient with hypothalamic hamartoma. J Neurosurg 89: 645–648
5. Barcia Salorio JL, Garcia JA, Hernandez G, Lopez Gomez L (1993) Radiosurgery of epilepsy: long-term results. Presented at the European Society for stereotactic and functional neurosurgery
6. Barcia Salorio JL, Roldan P, Hernandez G, Lopez Gomez L (1985) Radiosurgery treatment of epilepsy. Appl Neurophysiol 48: 400–403
7. Barcia Salorio JL, Vanaclocha V, Cerda M, Roldan P (1985) Focus irradiation in epilepsy. Experimental study in the cat. Appl Neurophysiol 48: 152
8. Bartolomei F, Regis J, Kida Y, Kobayashi T, Vladyka V, Liscak R, Forster D, Kemeny A, Shrotner O, Pendl G (1999) Gamma Knife radiosurgery for epilepsy associated with cavernous hemangiomas: a retrospective study of 49 cases. Stereotact Funct Neurosurg 72 [Suppl] 1: 22–28
9. Bartolomei F, Wendling F, Vignal J, Kochen S, Badier J, LeBouquin-Jeannes J, Bellanger J, Chauvel P (1999) Temporal Lobe Epilepsies: identification of subtypes using coherence analysis in Stereoelectroencephalography. Clin Neurophysiol 110: 1741–1754
10. Berkovic SF, Andermann F, Melanson D, Ethier RE, Feindel W, Gloor P (1988) Hypothalamic hamartoma and associated ictal laughter. Evolution of a characteristic epileptic syndrome and diagnostic value of magnetic resonance imaging. Ann Neurol 23: 429–439
11. Casazza M, Broggi G, Franzini A, Spreafico R, Bracchi M, Valentini M (1996) Supratentorial cavernous angiomas and epileptic seizures: preoperative course and post-operative outcome. Neurosurgery 39: 26–34
12. Chalifoux R, Elisevich K (1996) Effects of ionizing radiation on partial seizures attributable to malignant cerebral tumors. Stereotact Funct Neurosurg 67: 169–182
13. Cohen D, Zubay G, Goodman R (1995) Seizure outcome after lesionectomy for cavernous malformations. J Neurosurg 83: 237–242
14. Elwes R, Dunn G, Binnie C, Polkey C (1991) Outcome following resective surgery for temporal lobe epilepsy: a prospective follow up study of 102 consecutive cases. J Neurol Neurosurg Psychiatry 54: 949–952
15. Engel J (1996) Surgery for seizures. N Engl J Med 334: 647–652
16. Engel J, VanNess P, Rasmussen T, Ojemann L (1993) Outcome with respect to epileptic seizures. In: Engel J (ed) Surgical treatment of the epilepsies. Raven Press, New York, pp 609–622
17. French J, Williamson P, Thadani V, Darcey T, Mattson R, Spencer S, Spencer D (1993) Characteristics of medial temporal lobe epilepsy: I. Results of history and physical examination. Ann Neurol 34: 774–780
18. Giulinoni M, Acciari N, Padovani R, Galassi E (1995) Results of surgery in children with cerebral cavernous angiomas causing epilepsy. Br J Neurosurg 9: 135–141
19. Guldvog B, Loyning Y, Hauglie-Hanssen E (1991) Surgical versus medical treatment of epilepsy .I. Outcome related to survival, seizures and neurological deficit. Epilepsia 32: 375–388
20. Guldvog B, Loyning Y, Hauglie-Hanssen E (1991) Surgical versus medical treatment of epilepsy .II. Outcome related to social areas. Epilepsia 32: 477–486
21. Hayashi M, Bartolomei F, Rey M, Farnarier P, Chauvel P, Regis J (2002) MR changes after Gamma knife radiosurgery for Mesial Temporal Lobe Epilepsy: an evidence for the efficacy of subnecrotic doses. In: Kondziolka D (ed) Radiosurgery. Karger, Basel, pp submitted
22. Heikkinen ER, Konnov B, Melnikow L (1989) Relief of epilepsy by radiosurgery of cerebral arteriovenous malformations. Stereotact Funct Neurosurg 53: 157–166
23. Isnard J, Ryvlin P, Guenot M, Ostrowski K, Fisher C, Sindou M, Mauguiére F (1998) Role of the insular cortex in temporolimbic seizures: a stereo encephalographic (SEEG) study. Epilepsia 39 [Suppl] 6: 65
24. Kahane P, Munari C, Hoffmann D, Tassi L, Gallina P, Francione S, Di Leo M, Quarato P, Lo Russo G, Benabid A (1994) Approche chirurgicale multimodale des angiomes caverneux épileptogènes. Epilepsies 6: 113–130
25. Kahane P, Munari C, Minotti L, Hoffmann D, Tassi L, Pasquier B, Grand S, Benabid AL (1997) Role of the hypothalamic hamartoma in the genesis of gelastic and dacrystic seizures. In: Tuxhorn I, Holthausen H, Boenigk H (eds) Pediatric epilepsy syndromes and their surgical treatment. John Libbey, London, pp 447–461
26. Kahane P, Tassi L, Hoffmann D, Francione S, Gratadou-Jery G, Pasquier B, Munari C (1994) Crises dacrystiques et hamartome hypothalamique: à propos d'une observation vidéo-stéréo-EEG. Epilepsies 6: 259–279
27. Karlsson B, Kihlström L, Lindquist C, Ericson K, Steiner L (1998) Radiosurgery for cavernous malformations. J Neurosurg 88: 293–297
28. Kihlström L, Guo WY, Lindquist C, Mindus P (1995) Radiobiology of radiosurgery for refractory anxiety disorders. Neurosurgery 36: 294–302

29. Kondziolka D, Lunsford L, Flickinger J, Kestle J (1995) Reduction of hemorrhage risk after stereotactic radiosurgery for cavernous malformations. J Neurosurg 83: 825–831
30. Leksell L (1951) The stereotaxic method and radiosurgery of the brain. Acta Chir Scand 102: 316–319
31. Leksell L (1971) Stereotaxic radiosurgery in trigeminal neuralgia. Acta Chir Scand 137: 311–314
32. Leksell L (1971) Stereotaxis and radiosurgery. An operative system. Thomas CC, Springfield
33. Lindquist C, Kilström L, Hellstrand E (1991) Functional neurosurgery – A future for the Gamma Knife? Stereotact Funct Neurosurg 57: 72–81
34. Lindquist C, Steiner L, Hindmarsh T (1992) Gamma knife thalamotomy for tremor: Report of two cases. In: Steiner L (ed) Radiosurgery: baseline and trends. Raven Press, New York, pp 237–243
35. Lunsford LD (1990) Stereotactic radiosurgery of intracranial arteriovenous malformations. In: W RH, R SS (eds) Neurosurgery update. Mc Graw-Hill, New York, pp 175–185
36. Lunsford LD (1993) The future of Gamma Knife stereotactic radiosurgery. In: Alexander E, III, Loeffler JS, Lunsford LD (eds) Stereotact radiosurg. Mc Graw-Hill, New York, pp 235–242
37. Maesawa S, Kondziolka D, Dixon C, Balzer J, Fellows W, Lunsford L (2000) Subnecrotic stereotactic radiosurgery controlling epilepsy produced by kainic acid injection in rats. J Neurosurg 93: 1033–1040
38. Marraire JN, Awad IA (1995) Intracranial cavernous malformations: lesion behavior and management strategies. Neurosurgery 37: 605
39. Mori Y, Kondziolka D, Balzer J, Fellows W, Flickinger J, Lunsford L, Thulborn K (2000) Effects of stereotactic radiosurgery on an animal model of hippocampal epilepsy. Neurosurgery 46: 157–165; discussion 165–158
40. Munari C, Kahane P, Francione S, Hoffmann D, Tassi L, Cusmai R, Vigevano F, Pasquier B, Betti O (1995) Role of the hypothalamic hamartoma in the genesis of gelastic fits (a video-stereo-EEG study). Electroencephalogr Clin Neurophysiol 95: 154–160
41. Pendl G, Eder H, Schroettner O, Leber K (1999) Corpus callosotomy with radiosurgery. Neurosurgery 45: 303–307; discussion 307–308
42. Pilcher WH, Roberto DW, Flanigin HF, Crandall PH, Wieser HG, Ojemann GA, Peacock WJ (1993) Complications of epilepsy surgery. In: Engel J (ed) Surgical treatment of epilepsies. Raven Press, New York, pp 565–581
43. Porter P, Willinsky R, Harper W, Wallace M (1997) Cerebral cavernous malformations: natural history and prognosis after clinical deterioration with or without hemorrhage. J Neurosurg 87: 190–197
44. Regis J, Bartolomei F, de TB, Genton P, Kobayashi T, Mori Y, Takakura K, Hori T, Inoue H, Schrottner O, Pendl G, Wolf A, Arita K, Chauvel P (2000) Gamma knife surgery for epilepsy related to hypothalamic hamartomas. Neurosurgery 47: 1343–1351; discussion 1351–1342
45. Régis J, Bartolomei F, Hayashi M, Roberts D, Chauvel P, Peragut J (2000) Role of Gamma Knife surgery in the treatment of severe epilepsies. Epileptic Disorders
46. Régis J, Bartolomei F, Kida Y, Kobayashi T, Vladyka V, Liscàk R, Forster D, Kemeny A, Schröttner O, Pendl G (2000) Radiosurgery of Epilepsy Associated with Cavernous Malformation: Retrospective study in 49 patients. Neurosurgery 47: 1091–1097
47. Regis J, Bartolomei F, Metellus P, Rey M, Genton P, Dravet C, Bureau M, Semah F, Gastaut J, Peragut J, Chauvel P (1999) Radiosurgery for trigeminal neuralgia and epilepsy. Neurosurg Clin N Am 10: 359–377
48. Régis J, Bartolomei F, Rey M, Genton P, Dravet C, Semah F, Gastaut J, Chauvel P, Peragut J (1999) Gamma knife surgery for mesial temporal lobe epilepsy. Epilepsia 40: 1551–1556
49. Regis J, Bartolomei F, Rey M, Hayashi M, Chauvel P, Peragut J (2000) Gamma knife surgery for mesial temporal lobe epilepsy. J Neurosurg 93 [Suppl] 3: 141–146
50. Régis J, Bartolomei F, Rey M, Hayashi M, Genton P, Dravet C, Bureau M, Semah F, Gastaut J-L, Chauvel P, Peragut J-C (2000) Role of Gamma Knife Surgery in the Treatment of Severe Epilepsies. In: Wyllie E (ed) The treatment of epilepsy: principle and practice. William & Wilkins, Baltimore (in press)
51. Régis J, Kerkerian-Legoff L, Rey M, Viale M, Porcheron D, Nieoullon A, Peragut J-C (1996) First biochemical evidence of differential functional effects following gamma knife surgery. Stereotact Funct Neurosurg 66: 29–38
52. Régis J, Peragut J, Rey M *et al* (1994) First selective amygdalohippocampic radiosurgery for mesial temporal lobe epilepsy. Stereotact and Functional Neurosurg 64 [Suppl] 1: 191–201
53. Régis J, Peragut JC, Rey M, Samson Y, Levrier O, Porcheron D, Regis H, Sedan R (1994) First selective amygdalohippocampic radiosurgery for mesial temporal lobe epilepsy. Stereotactic and Functional Neurosurgery 64: 191–201
54. Régis J, Roberts D (1999) Gamma Knife radiosurgery relative to microsurgery: epilepsy. Stereotact Funct Neurosurg 72 [Suppl] 1: 11–21
55. Regis J, Semah F, Bryan R, Levrier O, Rey M, Samson Y, Peragut J (1999) Early and delayed MR and PET changes after selective temporomesial radiosurgery in mesial temporal lobe epilepsy. AJNR Am J Neuroradiol 20: 213–216
56. Rogers L, Morris H, Lupica K (1993) Effect of cranial irradiation on seizure frequency in adults with low-grade astrocytoma and medically intractable epilepsy. Neurology 43: 1599–1601
57. Rossi G, Scerrati M, Roselli R (1985) Epileptogenic cerebral low grade tumors: effect of interstital stereotactic irradiation on seizures. Appl Neurophysiol 48: 127–132
58. Rougier A, Dartigues J, Commenges D, Claverie B, Loiseau P, Cohadan F (1992) A longitudinal assessment of seizure outcome and overall benefit from 100 corticecomies for epilepsy. J Neurol Neurosurg Psychiatry 55: 762–767
59. Schröttner O, Pendl G, Unger F, Feichtinger K (1997) Radiosurgery in Lesional Epilepsy: Brain Tumors. Stereotactic and Functional neurosurgery 70 [Suppl] 1: 50–56
60. Seo Y, Fukupka S, Takanashi M, Nakagawara J, Suematsu K, Nakamura J, Nagashima K (1997) Gamma Knife surgery for angiographically occult vascular malformations. Stereotact Funct Neurosurg 64: 98–109
61. Spencer D, Inserni J (1991) Temporal lobectomy. In: Luders HO (ed) Epilepsy surgery. Raven Press, New York, pp 533–545
62. Spencer S (1996) Long term outcome after Epilepsy Surgery. Epilepsia 37: 807–813
63. Sperling M, O'Connor M, Saykin A (1995) Five year outcome of temporal lobectomy for refractory epilepsy. Neurology 45: 395
64. Steiner L, Forster D, Leksell L (1980) Gammathalamotomy in intractable pain. Acta Neurochir (Wien) 52: 173–184
65. Steiner L, Lindquist C (1987) Radiosurgery in cerebral arterioveinous malformation. In: T RR (ed) Neurosurgery: state of the art reviews, pp 329–335
66. Steiner L, Lindquist C, Adler J, Torner J, Alves W, Steiner M (1992) Clinical outcome of radiosurgery for cerebral arteriovenous malformations. J Neurosurg 77: 1–8
67. Talairach J, Bancaud J, Szikla G, Bonis A, Geler S, Vedrenne C (1974) Approche nouvelle de la neurochirurgie de l'epilepsie. Méthodologie stéréotaxique et résultats thérapeutiques. In:

Neurochirurgie (ed) Congrés Annuel de la Société de Langue Française. Marseille 25–28 Juin 1974, Masson, pp 205–213
68. Tassinari CA, Riguzzi P, Rizzi R, Passarelli D, Volpi L (1997) Gelastic Seizures. In: Tuxhorn I, Holthausen H, Boenigk H (eds) Current problems in epilepsy. John Libbey, London, pp 429–446
69. Weil S, Tew J, Steiner L (1990) Comparison of radiosurgery and microsurgery for the treatment of cavernous malformations of the brainstem. J Neurosurg 75: 32–39
70. Whang C, Kim C (1994) Short-term follow-up of stereotactic Gamma-Knife radiosurgery in epilepsy. Presented at the Leksell Gamma Knife Society, Kyoto, Japan
71. Whang CJ, Kwon Y (1996) Long-Term Follow-Up of Stereotactic Gamma Knife Radiosurgery in Epilepsy. Stereo Functional Neurosurg 66 [Suppl] 1: 349–356
72. Wieser H, Engel JJ, Williamson P, Babb T, Gloor P (1993) Surgically remediable temporal lobes syndromes. In: Jr JE (ed) Surgical treatment of the epilepsies, 2nd edn. Raven Press, New York, pp 49–63
73. Wieser HG (1984) Selective amygdalohippocampectomy as a surgical treatment of mediobasal limbic epilepsy. Surg Neurol 17: 445–457
74. Wieser HG, Siegel AM, Yasargil GM (1990) The Zurich amygdalo-hippocampectomy series: a short up-date. Acta Neurochir (Wien) [Suppl] 50: 122–127
75. Wilson W, Swartzwelder HS, Anderson WW, Lewis DV (1988) Seizure activity in vitro: a dual focus model. Epilepsy Res 2: 289–293
76. Wingkun EC, Awad IA, Lüders H, Awad CA (1991) Natural history of recurrent seizures after resective surgery for epilepsy. Epilepsia 32: 851–856
77. Young R, Vermelen SS, Grimm P, Posewitz AE, Jacques DB, Rand RW, Copcutt BG (1994) Gamma Knife thalamotomy for the treatment of persistant pain. Stereotactic and Functional neurosurgery 64 [Suppl] 1: 172–181
78. Zevgaridis D, Van Velthoven V, Ebelling U, Reulen H (1996) Seizure control following surgery in supratentorial cavernous malformations: a retrospective study in 77 patients. Acta Neurochir (Wien) 138: 672–677

Correspondence: Dr J. Régis, Service de Neurochirurgie Fonctionnelle et Stéréotaxique, C.H.U. La Timone, 264 rue Saint Pierre, 13385 Marseilles Cedex 05, France.

Acta Neurochir (2002) [Suppl] 84: 49–55

Gamma-Knife Radiosurgery of Mesiotemporal Tumour Epilepsy Observations and Long Term Results

O. Schröttner[1], **F. Unger**[1], **H. G. Eder**[1], **M. Feichtinger**[2], and **G. Pendl**[1]

[1] Department of Neurosurgery, Karl-Franzens University, Graz, Austria
[2] Department of Neurology, Karl-Franzens University, Graz, Austria

Summary

Purpose. The efficacy of radiosurgery in cases of mesiotemporal tumours associated with long standing epilepsy has not clearly been documented up to now. The authors present a retrospective analysis of 19 cases treated by Gamma-Knife radiosurgery (GKRS) for mesiotemporal tumour epilepsy.

Methods. Between 1992 and 1997 19 patients (12 male and 7 female) with a mean age of 31 years (5–72) and mesiotemporal tumour-induced epilepsy of a mean duration of 8.6 years (0.9–28) were treated by GKRS. All tumours were within the mesiotemporal structures and the pathohistology proven by biopsy or resective procedure revealed 15 (79%) low grade astrocytomas, 3 (16%) gangliogliomas and 1 (5%) cavernoma. Beside tumour control, the main aim of GKRS was alleviation of epilepsy by irradiating the presumed epileptic foci outside the tumour volume. The 50% isodose volumes surrounding the tumours measured a mean of 6.2 ccm (1.1–18 ccm). Doses given at marginal isodoses ranged from 12 to 30 Gy (mean 17.3 Gy). The outcome with respect to epileptic seizures was evaluated by the Engel classification.

Results. After a follow-up (FU) of 1.7 to 9.7 years (mean 6.5 years) 11 patients (57.9%) were significantly ameliorated (Engel I and Engel II), 7 patients (36.8%) worthwhile improved (Engel III) and 1 patient (5.3%) unchanged. In 11 patients (58%) radiosurgically induced image changes were seen on MRI.

Interpretation. Although microsurgical approach guided by electrocorticography (EcoG) is the state of art for treatment of mesiotemporal tumour epilepsy, GKRS can be used as a non-invasive, safe and effective alternative to resective surgery for selected cases.

Keywords: Mesiotemporal lobe epilepsy; Gamma-Knife radiosurgery; tumour epilepsy.

Introduction

The goals of radiosurgery (RS) for epilepsy associated with brain tumours are similar to those of epilepsy surgery for tumours, namely primary control of the tumour and reduction of seizure activity without associated neurologic morbidity.

Mesiotemporal lobe epilepsy is a very common, well characterized form of complex partial epilepsy (CPS). In mesiotemporal tumour epilepsy there is a complex relationship of the epileptogenic network in this region. From resective tumour epilepsy surgery in this location it is known that patients become less likely seizure free than after extratemporal resections.

Nevertheless in mesiotemporal tumour epilepsy Gamma-Knife radiosurgery represents a non-invasive method with the capabililty to control tumour-growth and epileptic activity.

Patients and Method

From July 1992 to July 1997, 19 patients (12 male and 7 female) with mesiotemporal tumour-induced epilepsy of a mean duration of 8.6 years (median 5 years, range 0.9–28 years) were treated with GKRS in our department. Patients' ages ranged from 5–72 years (mean 31 years, median 27 years). All patients had complex partial seizures, and in 11 of these there was secondary generalization. The neurological status revealed a slight hemiparesis in one patient and was normal in the others. The mean Karnofsky performance score was 90 (median 90, range 80–100). CT or MR imaging was performed in all patients. All tumours were within the mesiotemporal structures (amygdala, uncus, anterior and posterior hippocampus), 10 involving the right and 9 the left side. The histopathology had been proven by biopsy in 9 patients and by specimens of one to three resections in 10 patients. In 15 patients (79%) a low-grade astrocytoma (11 grade II astrocytomas, 3 oligoastrocytomas, 1 pilocytic astrocytoma) had been diagnosed. Other histopathologies had been 3 gangliogliomas and 1 cavernoma (Table 1).

All patients underwent preoperative interictal and ictal EEG-recording indicating an epileptic focus consistent with the tumour location. Beside tumour control, the main aim of radiosurgery was alleviation of epilepsy by irradiating the presumed epileptic foci outside the tumour volumes.

Therefore the intention of the treatment was to irradiate as large volumes of the mesiotemporal structure as possible outside the tumour volume. For the entire group, the 50% mean isodose volumes, which surrounded the tumour volumes, measured 6.2 ccm (median 5.2 ccm, range 1.1–18 ccm). Volumes of these isodoses were calculated using GammaPlan treatment planning system. In 7 patients

Table 1. *Patients Characteristics and Radiosurgical Treatment Parameters in 19 Patients with GKRS of Mesiotemporal Tumour Epilepsy*

No.	Sex	Age (yrs)	Seizure	Dur (yrs)	KPS	Hist	Lo	Pre OP	OP-GK (mo)	SV ccm	%	Dm Gy	MaxD Gy
1	m	24	CPS	3.50	90	Astro	l	B	1.4	4.7	50	20	40
2	m	22	CPS; G	16.00	100	Astro	l	B	0.6	12	40	15	37
3	f	25	CPS; G	18.00	90	Astro	r	R	5.5	13	50	30	60
4	f	27	CPS; G	27.00	90	Astro	r	R	15.7	5	50	20	40
5	m	34	CPS	1.00	90	OAstro	r	B	3.8	6.4	60	15	25
6	m	27	CPS	1.00	90	Cavern	l	B	0.8	3.6	50	16	32
7	f	14	CPS	5.00	90	Astro	l	R	8.4	5.6	50	17	34
8	m	72	CPS; G	1.50	90	Astro	l	R	0.9	3	50	20	40
9	m	65	CPS; G	1.00	90	Astro	l	B	1.2	4.1	30	12	40
10	m	19	CPS; G	12.00	90	Astro	r	R	42.3	18	60	13.5	22.5
11	f	18	CPS; G	17.00	90	G-Glio	r	R	3.5	2.4	50	15	30
12	f	5	CPS; G	5.00	80	OAstro	r	R	23.2	5.2	50	14	28
13	f	40	CPS	28.00	100	Astro	r	B	0.2	7.8	50	18	36
14	m	9	CPS	2.20	90	OAstro	l	R	26	4.8	60	15	25
15	m	16	CPS; G	1.20	100	G-Glio	r	B	0.03	1.1	45	12	26.7
16	m	27	CPS; G	2.30	80	Astro	l	R	26.5	5.6	50	12	24
17	f	46	CPS	5.00	100	Astro	r	B	2.3	7.4	50	25	50
18	m	36	CPS; G	15.00	80	G-Glio	r	R	89.8	6.9	50	25	25
19	m	66	CPS	0.90	100	PAstro	l	B	1	1.6	55	14	25.5

No. Number of the patient; *CPS* complex partial seizure; *G* generalization; *Dur* duration of epilepsy; *KPS* Karnofsky performance score; *Hist* pathohistology; *Astro* low-grade astrocytoma; *PAstro* pilocytic astrocytoma; *OAstro* oligoastrocytoma; *G-Glio* ganglioglioma; *Cavern* cavernoma; *Lo* side of tumour location; *Pre OP* preradiosurgical procedures; *B* biopsy; *R* resection; *OP-GK* time interval from Pre OP to GKRS; *SV* tumour surrounding isodose volume; % percentage of isodose lines; *Dm* dose at the margin; *MaxD* dose at maximum; *Gy* Gray.

with diffuse tumour spread larger volumes of the mesiotemporal structures had been included in the radiosurgical treatment volume (Table 1: cases No. 2–4, 10, 12–13, 16–17). Amygdala and the hippocampus had been included in the radiosurgical dose plan in one further patient with a residual small ganglioglioma of the uncus, where presurgical evaluation had shown mesiotemporal origin of the epilepsy (Table 1: case No. 18; Fig. 2).

For treatment the 201 source Gamma-Knife, Model B, was used. Doses given at a mean of 50% marginal isodose volumes (median 50%, range 30–60%) ranged from 12 to 30 Gy (mean 17.3 Gy, median 15 Gy). Doses at maximum ranged from 22.5 to 60 Gy (mean 32.7 Gy, median 32 Gy).

Outcome with respect to epileptic seizures was evaluated by the Engel classification [6], where class I is characterized as seizure free, class II as rare seizures (almost seizure free), class III as a worthwhile improvement and class IV as no worthwhile improvement.

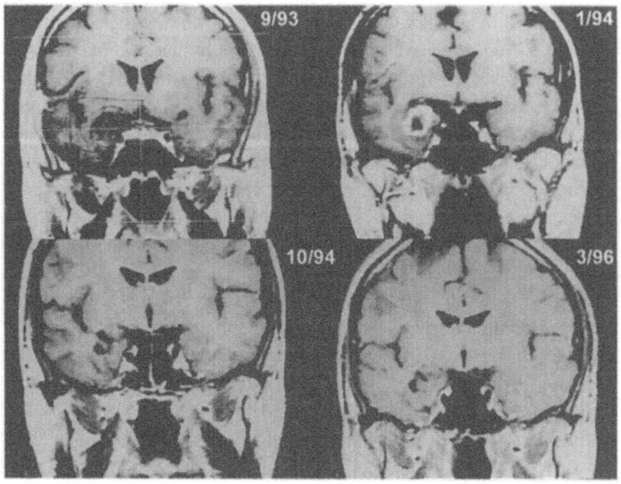

Fig. 1. *Case No. 5*: 34-year-old male presenting with CPS since 1 year. Biopsy of a small mass in the uncus revealed an oligoastrocytoma grade I. *9/93*: Dose plan at radiosurgery shows the 60% isodose volume surrounding the tumour. 15 Gy marginal dose had been applied (maximum dose 25 Gy). *1/94*: 4 months after GKRS a ring-shaped contrast enhancement is seen, corresponding to the 60% isodose volume. *10/94*: 9 months thereafter the contrast enhancement has disappeared, the tumour mass is reduced *3/96*: Stable situation of reduced tumour size 30 months after radiosurgery

Results

Imaging

In all patients, beside one patient in whome central tumour growth occurred, tumour control could be reached. A sudden onset of changes on the MRI with contrast enhancement corresponding to the tumour-surrounding isodose volume, occured in 11 patients (58%) after 3 to 30 months (mean 10.3 months, median 10 months). The 11 patients were treated with a mean isodose volume of 8 ccm (median 6.9 ccm, range 1.1–18 ccm), which is twice as large as the mean isodose volume of the other 8 patients, which measured a mean of 3.8 ccm (median 3.9 ccm, range 1.6–5.6 ccm). Doses given at the margin did not differ very much,

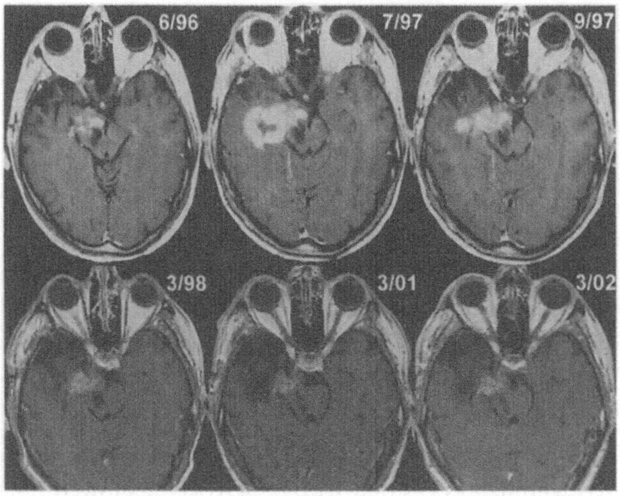

Fig. 2. *Case No. 18*: 36-year-old male. CPS with secondary generalization since 15 years. 2 times resection of a ganglioglioma. *6/96*: Preradiosurgical MRI showing residual tumour mass. *7/97*: 12 months after GKRS of tumour mass and mesiotemporal structures with an 50% isodose volume of 6.9 ccm and 25 Gy marginal dose. A contrast enhancement is seen corresponding to the 50% isodose volume. Patient experiences significant improvement of seizure activity. *9/97*: 2 months later the contrast enhancement is significantly smaller. *3/98*: contrast enhancement resolved 8 months after appearance. *3/01 and 3/02*: stable residual tumour mass 5.75 years and 6.75 years after radiosurgery

although they were higher in the "enhancement"-group with a mean of 18.7 Gy (median 17 Gy, range 12–30 Gy) in comparison to the other 8 patients with no image signs, who were treated with a mean of 15 Gy (median 15 Gy, range 12–20 Gy). This ring-shaped image change, with the aspect of a so called "radionecrosis", disappeared within 13 to 50 months (mean 27 months, median 23 months) after RS in 9 patients (Table 2; Fig. 2). In 2 patients (case No. 3 and No. 17), because of clinical signs of elevated intracranial pressure, postradiosurgical morphological change within mesiotemporal structures had been removed by open resection and been ascertained as radionecrosis by pathohistology.

Clinical Results

A reduction of seizure frequency and/or severity occured in 18 patients after 0.5 to 48 months (mean 9 months, median 4 months). Long term results after a FU time of 1.7 to 9.7 years (mean 6.5 years, median 6.7 years), including those 2 patients with resection of radionecrosis, revealed 11 patients (57.9%) significantly ameliorated (26.3% Engel I and 31.6% Engel II) and 7 patients (36.8%) worthwhile improved (Engel III). 2 patients died unrelated to radiosurgery 1.8 years (car accident) and 1.7 years (central tumour growth) after RS (case No. 8 and 16). Patient No. 6 had recurrent bleeding into the cavernoma without clinical signs and was operated 32 months after RS. Nevertheless this

Table 2. *Image Changes and Clinical Results after GKRS of Mesiotemporal Tumour Epilepsy*

No.	IM change (mo)	IM res (mo)	Clin (mo)	Engel class	FU (yrs)	KPS	Special outcome
1	8	30	24	III	9.7	90	–
2	4	46	–	IV	9.4	90	TLR after 51 mo
3	12	–	7	I	9.3	90	RN ex after 13 mo
4	–	–	48	III	8.7	90	–
5	4	13	14	II	8.5	90	–
6	–	–	3	II	7.3	90	R bleed cav after 32 mo
7	11	23	1	I	7.2	90	–
8	–	–	1	II	1.8	90	death after car accident
9	–	–	1	I	7.2	90	–
10	12	33	1	III	7.2	90	–
11	–	–	1	II	6.7	90	–
12	–	–	8	III	6.2	80	–
13	30	50	20	II	6.2	100	–
14	3	15	5	III	5.8	90	–
15	10	15	11	III	5.7	90	–
16	–	–	0.5	III	1.7	40	central tumour growth
17	7	–	3	I	5.2	100	RN ex after 10 mo
18	12	18	12	II	5.2	80	–
19	–	–	1	I	4.7	100	–

No. Number of the patient; *IM change (mo)* image change after (months); *IM res (mo)* image change resolved after (months); *Clin (mo)* first clinical results after (months); *FU* follow up time in (years); *KPS* Karnofsky performance score; *TLR* temporal lobe resection; *RN ex* extirpation of radionecrosis; *R bleed cav* resection of bleeding cavernoma.

patient was almost seizure-free from 3 months after RS to the 7.3 year FU time. One patient (5.3%) did not improve and was operated in another hospital 4.25 years after GKRS with temporal lobe resection without further clinical improvement.

There was no significant difference in outcome for the group with contrast enhancement at the border of the treatment volume (54.5% Engel I + II) in comparison to those patients without imaging changes (62.5% Engel I + II). With exception for patients No. 3 and 17, who experienced signs of elevated intracranial pressure for a short period of several days and for patient No. 16, whose general condition worsened due to central tumour growth, the postradiosurgical Karnofsky score remained the same and was a mean of 87.9 for all patients (median. 90, range 40–100).

Discussion

The way in which radiosurgery affects seizures can best be explained by the reports of Barcia *et al.* [2–3], who found that low doses of 10 to 20 Gy proved effective for epileptogenic activity supression. In his series, 82% of patients with electrocorticographically localized epileptic foci became seizure-free or had marked reduction of seizures. The effects were delayed in time and supported the hypothesis of long-term structural effect on the epileptic focus.

In lesional epilepsy the effect of GKRS is well documented for AVM patients with long standing seizure history: 51% to 60% of patients became seizure-free [16, 25].

Results of GKRS on tumour-induced epilepsy were reported by Whang *et al.* in 1995 [27]. His first report covered the short-term results with a mean FU time of 2.5 years (range 1.2–3.7 years) in 9 patients with epilepsy and nonprogressive cerebral lesions. The outcome was evaluated according to the Engel classification, and 90% of patients fell in class I or II. A second long term follow up report by Whang *et al.* in 1996 [28] deals with 23 patients and includes the 9 patients of the first report from 1995. Selection criteria were the same and observation times ranged from 1.2–4.5 years, with a mean FU time of 2.5 years. In this report only 56% of patients show favourable results of Engel class I or II. Interestingly, only those patients treated at times after the first report contributed to these worse results, while the good condition of those patients of the first report continued to be 90% in Engel I. Different factors influencing clinical outcome in the radiosurgical treatment of tumour-induced epilepsy are obvious.

Schröttner *et al.* 1997 [24] in a retrospective study analyse 26 patients with cerebral tumours – 65% were low-grade gliomas – and epilepsy which had been treated by radiosurgery for either reason. They found that GKRS could work if sufficient volume of brain tissue outside the tumour volume receives at least 10 Gy, which would support the observations of Barcia *et al.* [2–3]. The observations recorded in this study, although statistically insignificant due to the few numbers of cases, indicate that when a larger volume of brain outside the tumour receives at least 10 Gy the outcome is better.

A retrospective multicenter study of 49 patients with cavernomas associated with epilepsy [23] showed that 53% of patients with a mean FU 23.66 $\pm$ 13 months became completely seizure free with a mean delay of 4 months (median 6 months, range 0–9 months) after treatment. The mean dose at the marginal isodose volume was 19.17 $\pm$ 4.4 Gy. Cavernomas in the mesiotemporal region presented with a poor outcome of only 14% seizure free patients (Engel class IA) in comparison to the 69.5% seizure free patients with lesions in extratemporal location. This proved location as the most valuable prognostic factor for the outcome after GKRS in this entity. Furthermore this finding showed up the complex relationship of the epileptogenic network in the mesiotemporal region.

Gamma-Knife radiosurgery for mesiotemporal lobe epilepsy first had been performed 1993 in 4 patients with the Gamma-Knife and reported by Regis *et al.* in 1994 [20]. The indication for this non-invasive procedure had been seen the same as for selective amygdalahippocampectomy reported by Wieser *et al.* [29–30]. Two isocenters using an 18 mm collimator helmet had been focused to amygdala, hippocampal body, and the entorhinal area representing a 50% isodose volume of about 6.5 ccm. The delivered margin dose to the 50% isodose line was 25 Gy. Ten months control of MRI showed radical changes including contrast enhancement corresponding perfectly to the 50% isodose line, a low signal in T1 and a high signal in T2 images inside the target volume. Outside the target volume, oedema of the temporal white matter produced a mass effect and a shallow of the Sylvian fissure. The first patient in this series became seizure-free immediately and the second after a latency of almost 1 year. Reduced doses and target volumes in other patients resulted in a proportional decrease of the clinical results. At the time of this first report in 1994 there were only few reports considerating dose-volume relations in radiosurgery

[15, 7] and the optimum target, technical parameters and selection of patients had still to be defined. A multicenter study with a multidisciplinary prospective evaluation and treatment protocol was initiated and first results had been very reproducible after delivering a dose of 25 Gy at the 50% marginal isodose volume ranging from 6.5 to 7 ccm. Patients experienced a gradual decrease in frequency, intensity and duration of seizures. MR changes appeared with a median delay of 10.5 months (range 7–22 months). The onset of radiobiological changes was associated with headache, nausea and vomiting in 2 patients. This signs resolved immediately after prescription of low doses of steroids [21–22].

Nevertheless issues including dose selection and target volume necessary for a good clinical result, and the expected short and long term outcomes remain important for discussion in the scientific world [14]. Moreover dose-volume relations producing necrotizing versus non-necrotizing lesions have to be elucidated in the future. The mechanism of action and structural significance in non-necrotizing doses and volumes in mesiotemporal lobe radiosurgery remains unclear mainly in those cases where late disappearance of hyperintense T2 signal and ring-shaped contrast enhancement on MRI demonstrate intact radiosurgically treated targets.

Eleven patients in our mesiotemporal tumour epilepsy study developed imaging sign of a radionecrosis on MRI, with a ring-shaped contrast enhancement, corresponding to the margins of the treatment isodose volumes, after a mean of 10.3 months. In 2 of them because of clinical signs of elevated intracranial pressure this mesiotemporal volume had been resected and pathohistologically diagnosed as a radionecrosis. In all other 9 patients this image change resolved and was not seen any more on the MRI controls after a mean of 27 months. The 11 patients were treated with a mean isodose volume of 8 ccm (median 6.9 ccm, range 1.1–18 ccm), which is twice as large as the mean isodose volume of the other 8 patients, which measured a mean of 3.8 ccm (median 3.8 ccm, range 1.6–5.6 ccm). Doses given at the margin did not differ very much, although they were higher in the "enhancement"-group with a mean of 18.7 Gy (median 17 Gy, range 12–30 Gy) in comparison to the other 8 patients with no image signs, who were treated with a mean of 15 Gy (median 15 Gy, range 12–20 Gy). In case No. 3 a high marginal dose of 30 Gy was given at a large volume of 13 ccm: this explains the development of a radionecrosis sufficiently. Nevertheless the radionecrosis in case No. 17 with a volume of 7.4 ccm and a margin dose of 25 Gy, is in the range of the doses and volumes normally given for treating hippocampal sclerosis in patients with mesiotemporal epilepsy.

In case No. 18 normal mesiotemporal structures together with a residual ganglioglioma of the uncus invading into the cerebral peduncle had been radiosurgically treated with a volume of 6.9 ccm and with a 25 Gy marginal dose. Fig. 2 shows the sudden disappearance of image changes that may have been interpreted as "radionecrosis" at first.

The involvement of foreign tissue in a radiosurgical treatment volume may be of significant value for postradiosurgical tissue reaction. Low grade astrocytomas are diffusely infiltrating neoplasms and poorly demarcated. Therefore isodose volumes which seem to involve normal brain tissue may be infiltrated by tumour cells and the reaction to relatively low doses may be undue.

The patient presented in Fig. 1 with a relatively well demarcated oligoastrocytoma had been treated by the 50% isodose volume of 6.4 ccm and a relatively low dose of 15 Gy at the margin. A very sudden appearance of a typical ring-shaped contrast enhancement corresponding to the 60% isodsose lines shows the sensitive reaction of a tumour infiltrated tissue.

Explaining the role of radiosurgery for mesiotemporal lobe tumour epilepsy this new treatment has to be compared with the results of resective surgery. These results of resective epilepsy surgery for brain tumours are of course not transferable to GKRS for patients with tumour epilepsy. Nevertheless there are findings from which a lot can be learned.

The opinion of neurosurgeons about the extent of open resection is controversial. Some prefer to resect the tumour alone [1, 5, 9–10, 13], others advocate the use of intra- or extraoperative electrocorticography to guide their resections by detected epileptic foci [4, 12].

Goldring *et al.* in 1986 [10] analysed seizure outcome following surgery in 21 patients with chronic epilepsy and tumours with a FU of at least 1 year. 14 patients had lesion resection only and 7 had resection of the lesion and mesial temporal structures. Only 3 patients had further seizures, one in the lesion group and 2 in the lesion plus mesial structures group. The authors concluded that mesial resection was not necessary.

The reason for this observation may be that by the operative technique at that time complete tumour removal was associated with more retraction and pressure to brain tissue outside the tumour volume.

Cascino *et al.* 1992 [5] reported on the use of computer-assisted stereotactic lesionectomy in 23 patients. Theoretically this should best identify the lesion. 17 patients (74%) had a greater than 40% reduction in seizures, and 13 (56%) had an outcome Engel class I. Those with a temporal location were less likely to be seizure free, demonstrating the difficulty to treat this entity with favourable results.

Other authors conclude that, at least for temporal lobe tumours, there is a greater chance of becoming seizure free, when the epileptogenic region is removed. Jooma *et al.* 1995 [12] studied 30 patients with CPS and temporal lobe tumours comparing 16 patients with lesionectomies alone and 14 patients who had lesionectomies plus resection of the epileptogenic region identified by ECoG. 13 patients (92.8%) of the ECoG guided group became seizure free. In the group with lesionectomy alone this was the case in only 3 (18.75%) patients. Moreover, Pilcher *et al.* in 1993 [19] in a specific study of epileptogenic gangliogliomas found that in those patients with ECoG guided resections of a temporal lobe lesion the amygdala, hippocampus, and the gyrus parahippocampalis had been the actively discharging location, wheras no discharges came from the tumour associated cortex.

The overall result in our 19 patients show 59% of the patients significantly ameliorated supporting the observation of the results of Cascino *et al.* [5], although only 26.3% of patients became Engel I. This results resemble also that of Whang *et al.* [27–28] in an unselected group of tumour epilepsy patients. Our results are quite better than those with lesionectomies alone reported by Jooma *et al.* [12], where only 18.75% of patients became seizure free. The reason may be that a considerable volume in the mesiotemporal structures outside the tumour volume got sufficient doses of at least 10 Gy.

The disadvantage of GKRS in mesiotemporal tumour epilepsy is that intraoperative ECoG evaluation cannot be performed in a non-invasive procedure and that results occur after a delay of a mean of 9 months as seen in our study.

Some other factors influencing the clinical outcome have to be mentioned. One of them is pathohistology. The pathohistology in this study on mesiotemporal tumours revealed gangliogliomas, astrocytomas, oligoastrocytomas and one cavernoma. Gangliogliomas are solid, well circumscribed tumours, the majority are supratentorial, usually in the temporal lobe. Those are, although biologically indolent with anaplastic features restricted to the astrocytic component, associated with chronic epilepsy [11]. Low-grade astrocytomas are diffusely infiltrating neoplasms, most commonly seen in the cerebral hemispheres of young adults. The tumours are hence poorly demarcated and expand the affected part in the brain, blurring anatomical landmarks. Fibrillary astrocytomas, although histologically indolent, may progress to a higher grade of tumour. The overall 5-year survival rate is 27%. Nevertheless patients, in whom the sole presenting symptom was epilepsy, had a better prognosis with a 63% 5-year survival rate, unaffected by the time interval between the onset of seizures and the treatment by surgery [26]. Pilocytic astrocytoma WHO grade I is the most common glioma in children. The tumour is usually a well demarcated soft, gray mass and must be distinguished from fibrillary astrocytoma because of the uniformely better prognosis, with an overall survival of 82% at 10 and 20 years [8].

Oligoastrocytomas comprise both oligodendroglioma and astrocytoma. These tumours most commonly present with long-standing seizures. The prognostic significance is like an oligodendroglioma and less favourable than be thought having a 5 and 10 year survival rate of 75% and 46%, respectively.

Cavernomas of the mesiotemporal region present with poor outcome of only 14% seizure free patients and prove localization as the most valuable factor for outcome after GKRS for tumour epilepsy [23].

Another factor influencing clinical outcome may be the location of tumours in those cases where secondary epileptogenesis may occur. Indeed, failures of tumour epilepsy surgery can be correlated to the findings of Morrell *et al.* [17–18]. They found that approximately one-third of patients with tumour epilepsy develop secondary epileptic foci and continue to have clinical seizures after removal of the primary tumour lesion. Furthermore, Yeh *et al.* 1993 [31], in his series of surgically treated AVMs, found remote epileptic foci in the ipsilateral mesial temporal region. Furthermore the probability of occurence of these secondary foci is directly related to the duration of the illness [17].

Conclusion

If the results of GKRS in mesiotemporal tumour epilepsy are to approach the results of open epilepsy surgery, a relatively large volume and low-dose radiation must be applied outside the tumour volume. Nevertheless the preradiosurgical evaluation must be performed by all modern measures of epilepsy diagnosis and dose-volume relationships of GKRS have carefully to be considered. GKRS has the disadvantage lacking intraoperative ECoG evaluation; its advantage as a non-invasive method with no mortality and nearly no morbidity can be used as an alternative to resective surgery in mesiotemporal tumour epilepsy in selected cases where resections in eloquent regions failed to control tumour growth and epilepsy or where age and illness precludes open surgery.

References

1. Awad IA, Rosenfeld J, Ahl J, Hahn JF, Luders H (1991) Intractable epilepsy and structural lesions of the brain: mapping, resection strategies and seizure outcome. Epilepsia 32: 179–186
2. Barcia Salorio JL, Roldan P, Hernandez G, Lopez-Gomez L (1985) Radiosurgical treatment of epilepsy. Appl Neurophysiol 48: 400–403
3. Barcia Salorio JL, Barcia JA, Hernandez G, Lopez-Gomez L (1994) Radiosurgery of epilepsy. Long term results. Acta Neurochir (Wien) [Suppl] 62: 11–113
4. Berger MS, Ghatan S, Haglund MM, Dobbins J, Ojemann GA (1993) Low-grade gliomas associated with intractable epilepsy: seizure outcome utilizing electrocorticography during tumour resection. J Neurosurg 79: 69–79
5. Cascino GD, Kelly PJ, Sharbrough FW, Hulihan JF, Hirschorn KA, Trenerry MR (1992) Long-term follow-up of stereotactic lesionectomy in partial epilepsy: predictive factors and electroencephalographic results. Epilepsia 33: 639–644
6. Engel J Jr (1987) Outcome with respect to epileptic seizures. In: Engel J Jr (ed) Surgical treatment of the epilepsies. Raven Press, New York, pp 553–571
7. Flickinger JC, Lunsford LD, Kondziolka D (1991) Dose-volume considerations in radiosurgery. Stereotact Funct Neurosurg 57: 99–105
8. Forsyth PA, Shaw EA, Scheithauer BW, O'Fallon JR, Layton DD, Katzmann JA (1993) Supratentorial pilocytic astrocytomas. Cancer 72: 292–301
9. Fried I, Kim JH, Spencer DD (1994) Limbic and neocorical gliomas associated with intractable seizures: a distinct clinicopathological group. Neurosurgery 34: 815–824
10. Goldring S, Rich KM, Picker S (1986) Experience with gliomas in patients presenting with a chronic seizure disorder. Clin Neurosurg 33: 15–42
11. Johannsson JH, Rekate HL, Roessmann U (1981) Gangliogliomas: pathohistological and clinical correlation. J Neurosurg 54: 58–63
12. Jooma R, Yeh H, Privitera MD, Gartner M (1995) Lesionectomy versus electrophysiologically guided resections for temporal lobe tumours manifesting with complex partial seizures. J Neurosurg 83: 231–236
13. Kirkpatrick PJ, Honavar M, Janota I, Polkey CE (1993) Control of temporal lobe epilepsy following en bloc resection of low grade tumors. J Neurosurg 78: 19–25
14. Kondziolka D (1999) Functional radiosurgery. Topic review. Neurosurgery 44: 12–22
15. Lindquist C, Hindmarsh T, Kihlströhm L, Mindus P, Steiner L (1992) MRI and CT studies of radionecrosis development in the normal human brain. In: Steiner L *et al* (eds) Radiosurgery: baseline and trends. Raven Press, New York, pp 245–254
16. Lunsford LD, Kondziolka D, Flickinger JC, Bissonette DJ, Jungreis CA, Maitz AH, Horton JA, Coffey RJ (1991) Stereotactic radiosurgery for arteriovenous malformations of the brain. J Neurosurg 75: 512–524
17. Morrell F, Rasmussen T, Gloor P, De Toledo-Morrell L (1983) Secondary epileptogenic foci in patients with verified temporal lobe tumour. Electroencephalogr Clin Neurophysiol 56: 26P (Society Proceedings)
18. Morrell F, Wada J, Engel J Jr (1987) Appendix III: potential relevance of kindling and secondary epileptogenesis to the consideration of surgical treatment for epilepsy. In: Engel J Jr (ed) Surgical treatment of the epilepsies. Raven Press, New York, pp 701–707
19. Pilcher WH, Silbergeld DL, Berger MS, Ojemann GA (1993) Intraoperative electrocorticography during tumour resection: impact on seizure outcome in patients with gangliogliomas. J Neurosurg 78: 891–902
20. Regis J, Peragut JC, Rey M, Samson Y, Levrier O, Porcheron D, Regis H, Sedan R (1994) First selective amygdalohippocampic radiosurgery for mesial temporal lobe epilepsy. Stereotact Funct Neurosurg [Suppl] 1 64: 191–201
21. Regis J, Bartolomei F, Rey M, Genton P, Dravet C, Semah F, Gastaut J, Chauvel P, Peragut J (1999) Gamma knife surgery for mesial temporal lobe epilepsy. Epilepsia 40: 1551–1556
22. Regis J, Semah F, Bryan R, Levrier O, Rey M, Samson Y, Peragut J (1999) Early and delayed MR and PET changes after selective temporomesial radiosurgery in mesial temporal lobe epilepsy. Am J Neuroradiol 20: 213–216
23. Regis J, Bartolomei F, Kida Y, Kobayashi T, Vladyka V, Liscak R, Forster D, Kemeny A, Schröttner O, Pendl G (2000) Radiosurgery of epilepsy associated with cavernous malformation: retrospective study in 49 patients. Neurosurgery 47: 1091–1097
24. Schröttner O, Pendl G, Unger F, Feichtinger K (1997) Radiosurgery in lesional epilepsy: brain tumours. Stereotact Funct Neurosurg 70 [Suppl] 1: 50–56
25. Steiner L, Lindquist C, Adler JR, Torner JC, Alves W, Steiner M (1992) Clinical outcome of radiosurgery for cerebral arteriovenous malformations. J Neurosurg 77: 1–8
26. Van Veelen ML, Avezaat CJ, Kros JM, van Putten, Vecht C (1998) Supratentorial low-grade astrocytoma: prognostic factors, dedifferentiation, and the issue of early versus late surgery. J Neurol Neurosurg Psychiatry 64: 581–587
27. Whang CJ, Kim JJ (1995) Short-term follow-up of stereotactic Gamma Knife radiosurgery in epilepsy. Stereotact Funct Neurosurg 64 [Suppl] 1: 202–208
28. Whang CJ, Kwon Y (1996) Long term follow-up of stereotactic Gamma Knife radiosurgery in epilepsy. Sterotact Funct Neurosurg 66 [Suppl] 1: 349–356
29. Wieser HG, Yasargil MG (1984) Selective amygdalahippocampectomy as a surgical treatment of medobasal limbic epilepsy. Surg Neurol 17: 445–457
30. Wieser HG, Engel J, Williamson PD, Babb TL, Gloor P (1993) Surgically remediable temporal lobe syndromes. In: Engel J (ed) Surgical treatment of the epilepsies. Raven Press, New York, pp 49–63
31. Yeh HS, Tew JM Jr, Gartner M (1993) Seizure control after surgery on cerebral arteriovenous malformations. J Neurosurg 78: 12–18

Correspondence: Oskar Schröttner, M.D., Department of Neurosurgery, Karl-Franzens University, Auenbruggerplatz 29, A-8036 Graz, Austria.

Acta Neurochir (2002) [Suppl] 84: 57–63

Stereotactic Radiosurgery for Hypothalamic Hamartomas

F. Unger[1], **O. Schröttner**[1], **M. Feichtinger**[2], **G. Bone**[3], **K. Haselsberger**[1], and **B. Sutter**[1]

[1] Department of Neurosurgery, Karl-Franzens University, Graz, Austria
[2] Department of Neurology, Karl-Franzens University, Graz, Austria
[3] Department of Radiology, Karl-Franzens University, Graz, Austria

Summary

Hypothalamic hamartomas are nonneoplastic lesions often characterized by central precocious puberty and gelastic epilepsy. Due to the delicate location surgery is often unsuccessful and associated with considerable risks. In the presented series, Gamma Knife radiosurgery was applied.

Four cases (aged between 5–13 years) who presented with medically intractable gelastic epilepsy and increasing secondary generalization, abnormal behaviour and precocious puberty (3 cases) are reported. Hypothalamic hamartomas sized 11–17 mm had been diagnosed by MR imaging. Radiosurgical treatment was performed in general anaesthesia with margin doses of 12–14 Gy to the 50–90% isodoses covering volumes of 600–2300 mm^3. After follow-up periods of 12 to 68 months, a continuing decrease both in seizure frequency and intensity was noted (outcome according to Engel: II a (3 cases) and III a (1 case)). All patients are socially reintegrated. MR imaging did not reveal significant changes concerning the size of the lesions. Gamma Knife radiosurgery can be an effective and safe alternative treatment modality for HH capable of achieving good seizure control and improving behavioural disorders in selected cases.

Keywords: Epilepsy; hypothalamic hamartoma; precocious puberty; radiosurgery

Abbreviations

CT computerized tomography
EEG electroencephalography
FSH follicle-stimulating hormone
GH growth hormone
GnRH gonadotropin-releasing hormone
HH hypothalamic hamartoma
LH luteinizing hormone
LHRH LH-releasing hormone
MR magnetic resonance
PP precocious puberty
RS radiosurgery
TSH Thyroid-stimulating hormone

Introduction

HH is a rare congenital heterotopic lesion consisting of neuronal tissue originating in the region of the tuber cinereum. In most cases, such lesions are discovered during the work up for PP (a complex problem of either central or peripheral origin) or seizures. The typical appearance is that of a spherical mass of the midline, usually located below the tuber cinereum and sized between 0.5 and 4.0 cm, in most cases less than 1.5 cm. HH may either be pedunculated or sessile [30, 36]. So far, the mechanism provoking the above mentioned symptoms is not yet fully understood. Seizures occur more often in sessile tumours and may take the form of gelastic epilepsy characterized by brief episodes of clonic facial grimaces accompanied by bubbling or laughing noises. Usually they start in the early childhood, occur frequently and constitute an unfavourable prognostic sign. Often this type of epilepsy is accompanied by a progressive mental deterioration [9].

Since 1934 when the first case was described [12], over 90 cases have been reported in the literature. Previous treatment modalities include surgical removal which is still controversial due to the peculiarity of the lesion and may result in hypothalamic dysfunction and damage to the mammillary bodies. Stereotactic radiofrequency thermocoagulation was successful in four patients, thus confirming the feasibility of this treating modality [16, 18]. So far, RS treatment has been reported in several cases [4, 23, 27, 35]. For the patients presented here, RS was applied because surgery of these lesions harbours considerable risks owing to their incorporation with hypothalamic tissue and the patients' parents kept insisting on a non-invasive therapy after being informed on therapeutic alternatives.

Patients and Methods

Between 1994 and 2001 four patients with HH were treated with stereotactic RS using the 201-source cobalt-60 Gamma Knife at the

Table 1. *Clinical Data on Hypothalamic Hamartomas with Intractable Epilepsy Treated Radiosurgically*

Case	Sex	Age (years)	Clinical presentation	Age at seizure onset (years)	Follow-up period (months)	Valdueza (36) classification	Cessation of seizures (months)	Effect on PP	Outcome (Engel) (14)
G. J.	M	5	Gel, GTCS, PP, BehDis	2	24	II b	9	NoCh	I (Seiz & BehDis) (IIa)
K. S.	M	6	GTCS, Temp, BehDis	5	12	II b	10	–	I (Seiz & BehDis) (IIa)
E. T.	M	13	Gel, GTCS, PP, BehDis	2	60	II b	10	NoCh	I (Seiz & BehDis) (IIa)
H. E.	F	6	Gel, GTCS, PP, BehDis	4	78	II b	16	NoCh	SI (Seiz & BehDis) (IIIa)

* *Gel* Gelastic epilepsy; *GTCS* secondarily generalized tonic-clonic seizures; *Temp* temporal seizures; *BehDis* behaviour and/or mental disorders; *PP* precocious puberty; *I* improved; *SI* slightly improved; *Seiz* seizures; *NoCh* No Change.

Table 2. *Radiosurgical Data of Patients with HH*

Case	Isodose (Gy)	Isocentres (mm)	Marginal isodose	Target volume (ccm)	Tumour volume (ccm)	Tumour size (cm)	Dose at optic tract (Gy)
G. J.	14	3 (2 × 8, 1 × 14)	65%	1.6	1.3	1.4	9
K. S.	12	7 × 8	50%	2.3	1.9	1.7	9
E. T.	12	1 × 14	90%	0.97	0.97	1.3	8
H. E.	12	4 × 8	60%	0.6	0.48	1.1	6

University of Graz, Austria. The age of these patients ranged from 5–13 years (median 6 years). There were 3 male and 1 female patients. The median age at the time of seizure onset was 2 years. All patients suffered from intractable seizures (Tables 1, 2) with a median duration of epilepsy of 3 years. Diagnosis was based on MR examination and clinical evaluation. EEG-recordings including video-EEG were not conclusive. Neuropsychological studies assessed the mental status and endocrinological examinations revealed precocious puberty in three patients. All patients underwent the procedure in general anaesthesia. Stereotactic RS using 201-cobalt-60 Gamma Knife was performed with a median dose at the marginal isodose of 12–14 Gy on the 50–90% isodose. Optic pathways received less than 10 Gy. Follow-up examinations were performed 6-monthly and included MR, EEG, clinical (neurological and ophthalmological) and neuropsychological evaluations.

Results

While all patients exhibited improvement, none of them is seizure-free. Improvement was graded according to Engel II a in three and III a in one patient [14]. Seizure improvement showed a median latency of 10 months (range: 9–16 months). Generalized seizures showed earlier and lasting cessation than gelastic ones. Behavioural disorders improved slightly according to neuropsychological testing. Actually all patients are socially integrated. Antiepileptic drugs were reduced in all patients. Unfortunately, the parents of the patient who had only slight improvement had not adhered strictly to the prescribed regimes.

After a mean time of 43 months (range: 12–78 months) no significant side effects (oedema or signs of intracranial hypertension) were reported. No optic tract deficits were discovered. No significant endocrinologic changes were noted. There was no impact on PP. The size of HH remained unchanged.

The following description of the radiosurgical outcome of a 15-year-old boy should demonstrate that seizure control and improvement of behavioural disorders can be achieved.

A presently 15 year-old boy was normal at birth. By the age of two years a gelastic epilepsy associated with a retardation in speech and motor activity emerged. Neurological and EEG examinations were not conclusive. Due to a suspected hearing loss the child underwent an ENT examination which resulted normal. Physical and mental development remained delayed. Since the age of 6 years, frequency and intensity of the gelastic seizures increased gradually and secondary generalization occurred. An interictual EEG examination demonstrated slow waves in the right temporal region, ictual EEG during gelastic seizures showed initially slow waves followed by diffuse depression and spike-waves. CT scans were not conclusive. At the age of 8 years a PP became evident, serum testosterone (6.1 ng/ml), LH-RH (9.7 mIU/ml) and LH (9.7 mIU/ml) corresponding to levels normally found in adults. GH and TSH were normal.

MRI studies carried out thereafter revealed a sessile HH (Fig. 1a), however, the boy's parents were reluc-

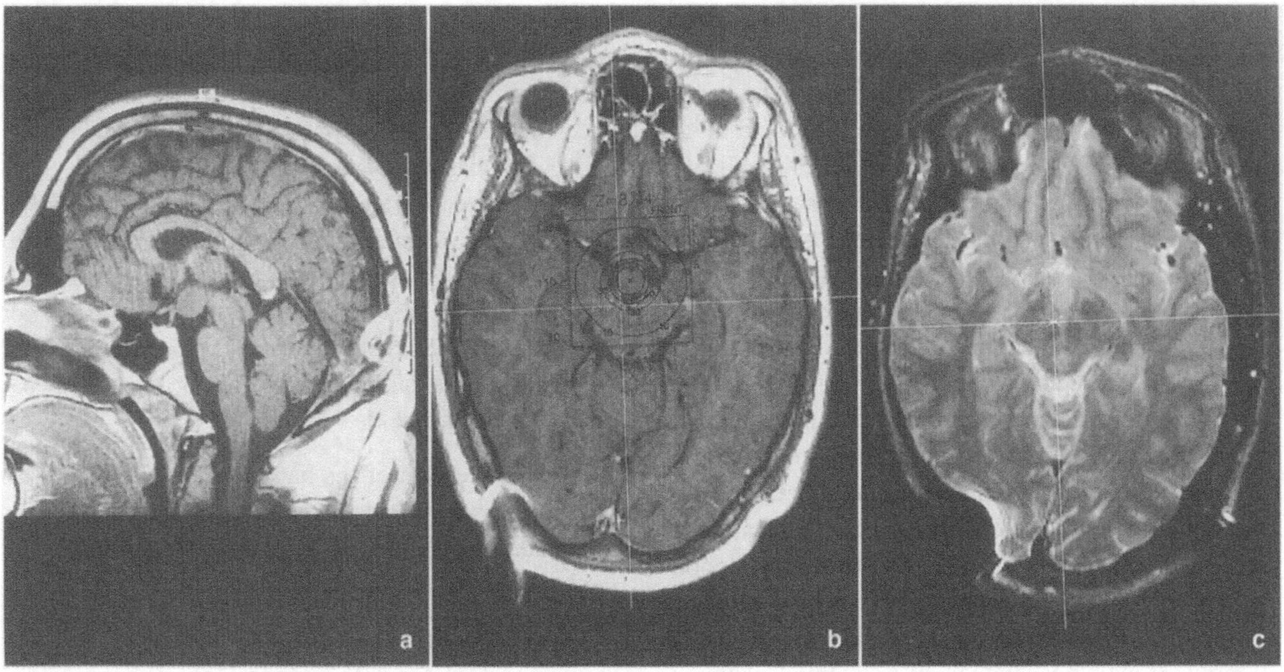

Fig. 1. Case T. E.: (a) T-1-weighted sagittal MR image with Gadolinium of a 13-year-old boy with a sessile HH measuring 13 mm in diameter which appears isointense in relation to gray matter before radiosurgery. (b) T-1-weighted axial MR image with Gadolinium for Gamma Knife planning. (c) T-2-weighted axial MR image for Gamma Knife planning demonstrates increased signal intensity

tant to any form of surgical intervention. At the age of 10 years the child was presented at our department for the first time with weight and height ranging beyond the 97th percentile. Within the following 3 years the boy became increasingly socially disabled because of a secondary generalization of seizures exceeding a frequency of 10 times a month accompanied by more than 50 gelastic seizures within the same period. As multiple drug regimes failed to achieve seizure control (last medication: Carbamazepine 1200 mg, Lamotrigin 200 mg) the patient was not able to attend school any longer. In January 1994, at the age of 13, the boy underwent Gamma Knife RS. The procedure was performed with the Leksell Gamma Knife Modell B using 201 Cobalt-60 beams delivering the irradiation. Equiped with an image-compatible Leksell stereotactic coordinate frame (Fig. 1b, 1c), the patient underwent the procedure in general anaesthesia. One shot with a marginal isodose volume of 12 Gy on the 90% isodose was applied through a 14 mm collimator with a target volume of 700 mm^3. The optic tract was exposed to an irradiation dose of 6 Gy in a very limited sector. The postradiosurgical course was uneventful. With a simultaneous improvement in social behaviour, epileptic activity began to decrease after one year. Neuroophthalmologic examination resulted normal. The results of hormonal studies were essentially the same as those obtained before radiosurgery with adult levels of serum testosterone, LH-RH, and LH. According to follow-up MR images there was no significant change in the size of the lesion. After a follow-up of 68 months the patient experienced only occasional gelastic seizures (less than 3 per month) but was free from generalized seizures, a daily dose of Carbamazepine of 900 mg as antiepileptic medication being tolerated well (Engel: IIa) [14]. Socially re-integrated, the boy has completed a basic school training. EEG findings improved, presently demonstrating only occasional slow waves on the right temporal side.

Discussion

There are recent reports providing encouraging evidence that RS may be safe and effective for treatment of intractable epilepsy due to HH [4, 27, 35].

Tuber cinereum is a descriptive name for the region including the small bilateral protuberances of gray matter and the middle hypothalamic nuclei located between the infundibular stalk and the large prominent mammillary bodies [10].

HH are congenital and thus do not represent true neoplasms. Developmentally, the tissue displacement probably arises when the ventral aspect of the neuroaxis is approaching the anterior tip of the end of the notochord in the 5th or 6th week of fetal life [8]. HH are characterized by a lack of invasiveness and stability in size over time. Both CT and MRI are invaluable in differentiating them from other suprasellar mass lesions in children. Craniopharyngiomas are often cystic, contain calcification and are rarely located isolated to the interpeduncular cistern. They may present a broad variety of appearances on MRI. Optic gliomas are mostly hypointense on T-1 and hyperintense on T-2-weighted images. In many cases, an enlargement of the optic nerves, optic chiasm or optic tract is to be seen. Intracranial germinomas constitute rare lesions enhancing on the application of contrast medium. Commonly, PP is not a typical clinical feature whereas tumour growth documented by sequential examinations supports the diagnosis of germinoma. Hypothalamic gliomas and gangliogliomas appear inhomogeneous and show contrast enhancement.

In HH, MRI studies show a mass isointense with gray matter and mostly hyperintense signal characteristics on T-2-weighted images [5, 11, 17]. MRI offers the additional advantage of an evaluation of any associated intracranial abnormalities like callosal agenesis, optic malformation, and hemispheric dysgenesis (heterotopias and microgyria) [8].

Valdueza *et al.* proposed a classification of HH based on topographical and clinical data from 42 patients. Based on the criteria size, type of attachment, origin, extent of hypothalamic displacement and common features four subgroups were established [36]. The patients presented in this paper meet the properties of Type II b (medium-large size, sessile with hypothalamic displacement, precocious puberty (3 cases), gelastic epilepsy, behaviour disorder).

The pathogenesis of PP remains uncertain. The mean age for onset of puberty is 10 years in girls and 12 years in boys, respectively, with a range of about 2 years. PP is diagnosed when typical signs occur in girls aged less than 8 years or in boys aged less than 9.5 years. A central PP is characterized by pubertal or adult levels of LH, FSH and estradiol or testosterone, and pubertal or mature responses to GnRH stimulation.

PP may arise following a stimulation of the anterior hypothalamus that is responsible for sexual development or in the posterior hypothalamus by mechanical interruption of inhibitory pathways to the pituitary gland locking the release of gonadotropin-releasing factor from the median eminence. In addition, a third mechanism with autonomous production and release of LH-RH has been suspected.

In our patients, precocious puberty was not resolved by RS. However, symptoms slowed down at least with respect to a decrease in serum levels of LH and FSH. An effect on seizures was observed delayed and did not correlate with changes in hormonal parameters.

Hypotheses explaining the origin of seizures in patients with HH include

a) interconnection of the hamartomous neurons with those of the limbic system or
b) seizures associated with midline abnormalities or hemispheric malformations.

Gelastic epilepsy is distinguished from epileptic laughter associated with temporal lobe seizures by onset, frequency and character [3, 9, 15, 18, 20, 21, 24, 25, 34]. The mechanism is unclear, representing either mechanical stimulation of the floor of the third ventricle by the tumour with epileptic discharge from the hypothalamus or some kind of automatism or release phenomenon. Temporal lobe epilepsy can also be associated with laughter. In the cases presented here, standard EEG was not able to detect the focus. Thus MRI studies were used for target localization.

Although epilepsy did not cease completely in the cases described above, there was a marked improvement in three cases and a worthwhile alleviation in one case.

Medication, surgery and radiotherapy have been used as treatment modalities in patients with HH. Long acting GnRH analogues have been effective in some cases, however, long term treatment is expensive.

Despite some reports of successful surgical treatment [1, 21, 28, 29, 36], surgery for HH has often been disappointing up to recent times [2, 11, 32]. Whereas asymptomatic HH would not require treatment at all, Valdueza recommends nevertheless surgery as therapy of choice in case of progressive visual impairment and failure of medical treatment (long-acting LHRH analogues) [36]. The same applies to patients with Type IIb hamartomas in whom epileptic activity and behavioural abnormalities are usually progressive and difficult to control. By contrast, Humphreys emphasizes the lack of extensive experience with treatment techniques for HH and remains uncertain about the benefit of exploration by open craniotomy [18]. The cur-

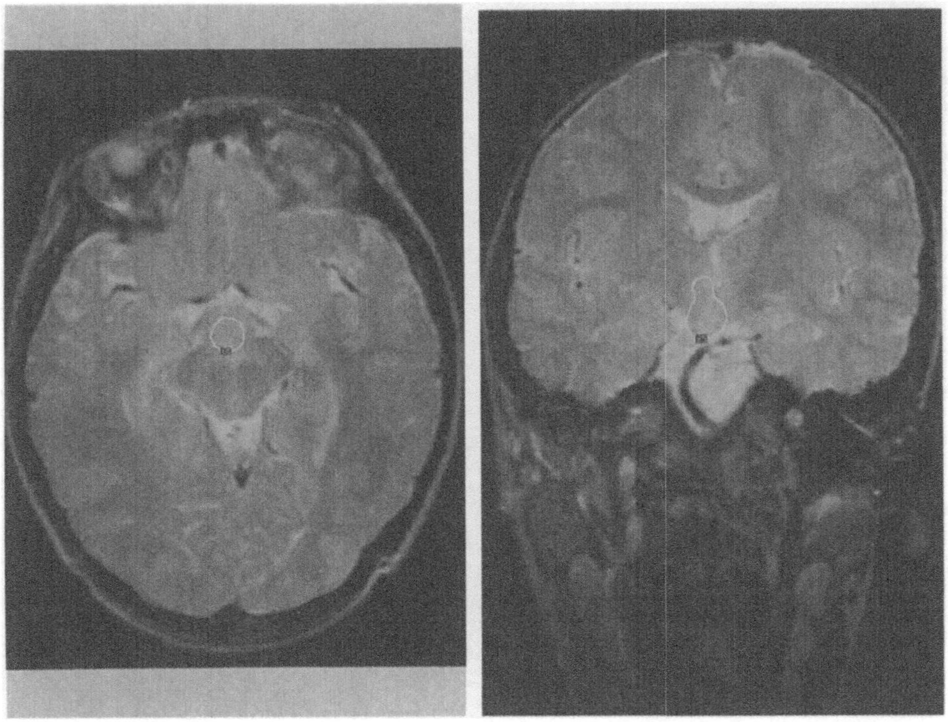

Fig. 2. Case G. J.: T-2 weighted coronal and axial MR images with Gadolinium of a HH for Gamma Knife planning displaying the 65% isodose (14 Gy)

rent opinion of surgical treatment of HH is formidable and complete excision is not technically achievable.

Being regarded as not radiosensitive, conventional radiotherapy has been rarely applied for hamartomas [29]. However, there are recent reports of successful stereotactic radiofrequency thermocoagulation. Kuzniecky *et al.* documented three cases of lesioning in HH with gelastic epilepsy [20], another one was reported by Fukuda *et al.* [16]. Seizures ceased according to depth electrode recording that allowed both a direct confirmation of the seizure focus and a guided placement of the electrodes. In contrast to RS, tissue samples for histological specification could be obtained.

There are various attempts to explain how RS may have a beneficial effect on epilepsy, yet the mechanism remains still uncertain [6, 19, 22, 27, 31, 35]. Understanding is limited with regard to the effects of RS on epileptic brain tissue. The mechanism of post-RS amelioration of epilepsy may be suppression of epileptogenesis (with low doses of radiaton) or destruction of pathways for the spread of epileptic activity as well as destruction of the epileptic focus (with high doses). Optimally, one would like to use non-necrotizing lower doses to effectively treat epilepsy and spare normal brain function. If there is a certain optimal radiation dose to prevent the epileptic focus from generating epileptic signals or to dissociate it from conducting signals without impairing normal function, RS may be an excellent way to control epilepsy. In patients with persistent seizures after a resection, RS could be used as an effective second-step approach to affect residual epileptogenic tissue. Based on experimental studies, Barcia Salorio *et al.* reported a hypothesis suggesting that there may be a decrease of gliosis in the focus responsible for a direct effect on pathological neurons [6].

Mori *et al.* developed a rat model of kainic acid-induced epilepsy to observe these effects and are still conducting their studies. Actually, they do believe in a positive effect of RS, but are reluctant until dose-response relationship is better characterized [22].

In some cases, RS in tumour-induced epilepsy may yield similar results as open epilepsy surgery, if a low-dose irradiation is applied to a relatively large volume outside the tumour volume. In our patients highly vulnerable structures in the hypothalamus had to be preserved. The marginal isodose of 12 Gy applied to the tumour had therefore to be delivered using an isodose configuration with a steep dose decline outside the tumour volume (Figs. 2, 3). The optic tract toler-

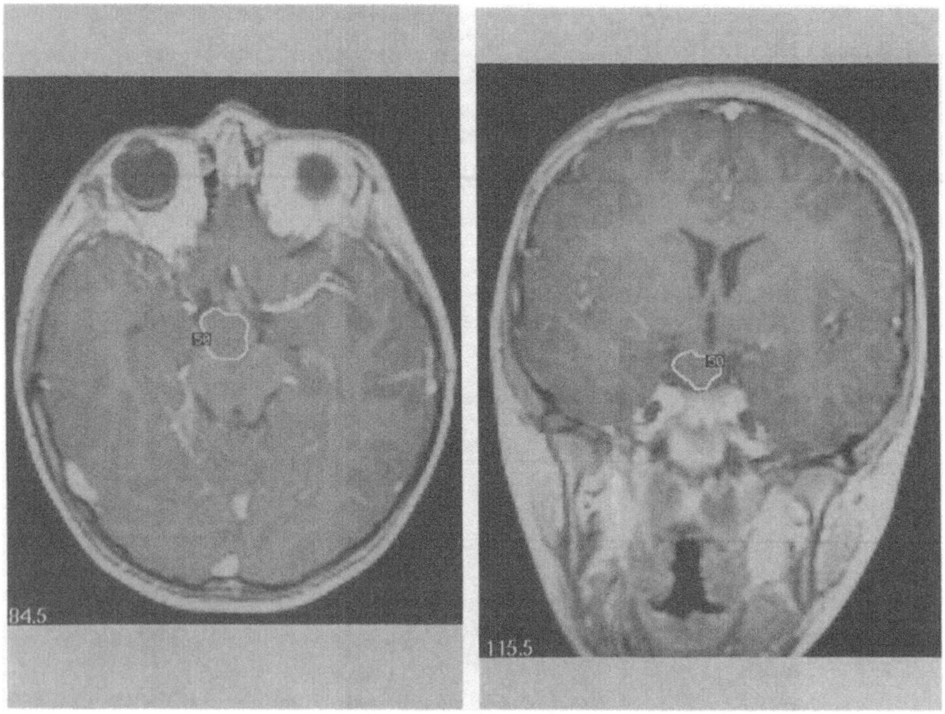

Fig. 3. Case K. S.: T-1 weighted axial and coronal MR images with Gadolinium of a HH for Gamma Knife displaying the 50% isodose (12 Gy)

ating up to 10 Gy was exposed to an irradiation dose of 6–9 Gy [19, 27]. Effects on epileptic activity that occurred progressively and delayed in time support the hypothesis of a long term structural change effecting the epileptogenic focus. Another case has recently been published by Arita *et al.* who stated that by a dose of 18 Gy to the 50% isodose seizure control was achieved and, moreover, a complete disappearance of the lesion was noted on MR images 12 months thereafter – a result that has to be regarded as extremely uncommon [4]. By contrast, Munari *et al.* reported a case in whom stereotactic RS by a linear accelerator proved to be ineffective. The authors attributed this unfavourable outcome to an inadequate dose-target relation [23].

Regis *et al.* recently reported several cases of HH treated successfully at a number of Gamma Knife centres. However, follow-up in his series is still short and he admits difficulties in accurately defining uniform standards. Some failures may be related to these errors [27].

Especially in children irradiation to the brain may give rise to severe side effects. Therefore also the option for Gamma Knife treatment has to be handled carefully. There are some reports about the role of radiosurgery in children [7, 13, 26]. While there are no long term follow-up examinations available so far, treatment has usually been well tolerated. Problems comparable to those observed after conventional external beam irradiation have not been noted. Mainly because of the necessity to immobilize the head in a stereotactic frame, children undergoing stereotactic radiosurgery frequently require general anaesthesia [33].

Conclusion

The application of RS in the treatment of intractable epilepsy is a relatively new and intriguing concept. Low irradiation doses (10–20 Gy) have proved effective for the suppression of epileptogenic activity and minimize the risk of complications due to irradiation toxicity. So far, the number of radiosurgically treated cases is still too small for final conclusions to be drawn and longer term outcomes are needed. This applies especially to children with precocious puberty in whom serum hormone levels did not return to normal range although an amelioration could be observed. Currently, radiosurgery for epilepsy is still looking for an optimization in the selection of irradiation dose, localization and target volume. None of the RS treatments approach the results of surgery in mesial temporal lobe epilepsy, for example.

Therefore RS may only be considered an alternative in cases with foci located close to functionally important brain areas because of a low risk of side effects.

Acknowledgment

We appreciate the sophisticated work of Ms Elfriede Meier in preparing the manuscript.

References

1. Albright AL, Lee PA (1993) Neurosurgical treatment of hypothalamic hamartomas causing precocious puberty. J Neurosurg 78: 77–82
2. Alvarez-Garijo JA, Albiach VJ, Vila MM *et al* (1983) Precocious puberty and hypothalamic hamartoma with total recovery after surgical treatment. Case report. J Neurosurg 58: 583–585
3. Ames FR, Enderstein O (1980) Gelastic epilepsy and hypothalamic hamartoma. S Afr Med J 58: 163–165
4. Arita K, Kurisu K, Iida K *et al* (1998) Subsidence of seizure induced by stereotactic radiation in a patient with hypothalamic hamartoma. Case report. J Neurosurg 89: 645–648
5. Arita K, Ikawa F, Kurisu K *et al* (1999) The relationship between magnetic resonance imaging findings and clinical manifestations of hypothalamic hamartoma. J Neurosurg 91: 212–220
6. Barcia Salorio JL, Barcia JA, Hernandez G *et al* (1994) Radiosurgery of epilepsy. Long-term results. Acta Neurochir (Wien) [Suppl] 62: 111–113
7. Bauman GS, Wara WM, Larson DA *et al* (1996) Gamma Knife radiosurgery in children. Pediatric Neurosurg 24: 193–201
8. Beningfield SJ, Bonnici F, Cremin BJ (1988) Magnetic resonance imaging of hypothalamic hamartomas. Br J Radiol 61: 1177–1180
9. Berkovic SF, Andermann F, Melanson D *et al* (1988) Hypothalamic hamartomas and ictal laughter: evolution of a characteristic epileptic syndrome and diagnostic value of magnetic resonance imaging. Ann Neurol 23: 429–439
10. Boyko OB, Curnes JT, Oakes WJ *et al* (1991) Hamartomas of the tuber cinereum: CT, MR, and pathologic findings. AJNR 12: 309–314
11. Burton EM, Ball WS Jr, Crone K *et al* (1989) Hamartoma of the tuber cinereum: a comparison of MR and CT findings in four cases. AJNR 10: 497–501
12. Chen TC, Gonzalez-Gomez I, McComb JG (1995) Uncommon glial tumors. In: Kaye AH, Laws ER (eds) Brain tumors. An encyclopedic approach. Churchill Livingstone, Edinburgh, pp 551–557
13. Eder HG, Leber KA, Eustacchio S, Pendl G (2001) The role of Gamma Knife radiosurgery in children. Childs Nerv Syst 17: 341–346
14. Engel J Jr (1987) Outcome with respect to epileptic seizures. In: Engel J Jr (ed) Surgical treatment of the epilepsies. Raven Press, New York, pp 553–571
15. Engelborghs S, Marien P, De Deyn P (2000) Gelastic epilepsy caused by hypothalamic hamartoma. Lancet 356: 940
16. Fukuda M, Kameyama S, Wachi M *et al* (1999) Stereotaxy for hypothalamic hamartoma with intractable gelastic seizures: technical case report. Neurosurgery 44: 1347–1350
17. Hahn FJ, Leibrock LG, Huseman CA *et al* (1988) The MR appearance of hypothalamic hamartoma. Neuroradiology 30: 65–68
18. Humphreys RP (1999) Stereotaxy for hypothalamic hamartoma with intractable gelastic seizures: technical case report. Neurosurgery 44: 1350 (Letter)
19. Kondziolka D (1999) Functional radiosurgery. Neurosurgery 44: 12–22
20. Kuzniecky R, Guthrie B, Mountz J *et al* (1997) Intrinsic epileptogenesis of hypothalamic hamartomas in gelastic epilepsy. Ann Neurol 42: 60–67
21. Machado HR, Hoffmann HJ, Hwang PA (1991) Gelastic seizures treated by resection of a hypothalamic hamartoma. Childs Nerv Syst 7: 462–465
22. Mori Y, Kondziolka D, Balzer J *et al* (2000) Effects of stereotactic radiosurgery on an animal model of hippocampal epilepsy. Neurosurgery 46: 157–168
23. Munari C, Kahane P, Francione S *et al* (1995) Role of the hypothalamic hamartoma in the genesis of gelastic fits (a video-stereo-EEG study). Electroencephalogr Clin Neurophysiol 95: 154–160
24. Pendl G (1975) Gelastic epilepsy in tumors of the hypothalamic region. In: Penholz H, Brock M, Hamer J *et al* (eds) Advances in neurosurgery 3. Springer, Berlin Heidelberg New York Tokyo, pp 442–449
25. Penfold JL, Manson JI, Caldicott WM (1978) Laughing seizures and precocious puberty: Case report and review of the literature. Aust Paediatr J 14: 185–190
26. Pollack IF, Albright AL (1996) Management of pediatric brain tumors. Neurosurg Q 6: 116–136
27. Regis J, Bartolomei F, Toffol BD *et al* (2000) Gamma Knife surgery for epilepsy related to hypothalamic hamartomas. Neurosurgery 47: 1343–1352
28. Rosenfeld JV, Harvey AS, Wrennall J *et al* (2001) Transcallosal resection of hypothalamic hamartomas, with cessation of seizures, in children with gelastic epilepsy. Neurosurgery 48: 108–118
29. Sato M, Ushio Y, Arita N *et al* (1985) Hypothalamic hamartoma: report of two cases. Neurosurgery 16: 198–206
30. Schiffer D (1997) Hamartoma of the hypothalamus. In: Schiffer D (ed) Brain tumors. Springer, Berlin Heidelberg New York Tokyo, pp 465
31. Schröttner O, Eder HG, Unger F *et al* (1998) Radiosurgery in lesional epilepsy: brain tumors. Stereotact Funct Neurosurg 70 [Suppl 1]: 50–56
32. Starceski PJ, Lee PA, Albright AL *et al* (1990) Hypothalamic hamartomas and sexual precocity. Evaluation of treatment options. AM J Dis Child 144: 225–228
33. Stokes MA, Soriano SG, Tarbell NJ *et al* (1995) Anesthesia for stereotactic radiosurgery in children. J Neurosurg Anesthesiol 7: 100–108
34. Striano S, Meo R, Bilo L *et al* (1999) Gelastic epilepsy: Symptomatic and cryptogenic cases. Epilepsia 40: 294–302
35. Unger F, Schröttner O, Haselsberger K *et al* (2000) Gamma knife radiosurgery for hypothalamic hamartomas in patients with medically intractable epilepsy and precocious puberty. Report of two cases. J Neurosurg 92: 726–731
36. Valdueza JM, Cristante L, Dammann O *et al* (1994) Hypothalamic hamartomas: With special reference to gelastic epilepsy and surgery. Neurosurgery 34: 949–958

Correspondence: Frank Unger, M.D., Department of Neurosurgery, Karl-Franzens University, Auenbruggerplatz 29, 8036 Graz, Austria.

Acta Neurochir (2002) [Suppl] 84: 65–70

Fractionated Stereotactically Guided Radiotherapy of Pharmacoresistant Temporal Lobe Epilepsy

G. G. Grabenbauer[1], Ch. Reinhold[1], F. Kerling[3], R. G. Müller[2], U. Lambrecht[1], E. Pauli[3], O. Ganslandt[4], R. Sauer[1], and H. Stefan[3]

[1] Department of Radiation Therapy, Erlangen, Germany
[2] Department of Medical Physics, Erlangen, Germany
[3] Division of Epileptology of the Department of Neurology, Erlangen, Germany
[4] Department of Neurosurgery, Friedrich-Alexander University of Erlangen-Nürnberg, Erlangen, Germany

Summary

Purpose. This prospective study evaluated the efficacy of fractionated stereotactically guided radiotherapy (SRT) as a treatment of pharmacoresistant temporal lobe epilepsy.

Patients and Methods. Inclusion criteria were patients aged between 17 and 65 years with unilateral temporal focus, without sufficient epilepsy control by antiepileptic drugs or neurosurgery. Two groups of 6 patients each were treated with 21 Gy (7 times 3 Gy) and 30 Gy (15 times 2 Gy). Study end points were change in seizure frequency, intensity, seizure length and neuropsychological parameters.

Results. All patients experienced a marked reduction in seizure frequency. The mean reduction of seizures was 37% (range 9–77%, i.e. seizures reduced from a monthly mean number of 11.75 to 7.52) at 18 months following radiation treatment and 46% (23–94%, i.e. 0.2–23 seizures per month) during the whole follow-up time. Seizure length was reduced in 5 out of 11 patients and intensity of seizures in 7 out of 11 patients.

Conclusion. Radiotherapy was identified as a safe and effective treatment for pharmacoresistant epilepsy since a good reduction of seizure frequency during longer follow-up was observed. SRT means an appropriate alternative for patients with contraindication against neurosurgery or insufficient seizure reduction after neurosurgery.

Keywords: Fractionated stereotactic radiotherapy; pharmacoresistant temporal lobe epilepsy.

Introduction

Pharmacoresistant epilepsy is invariably associated with a considerable loss of quality of life. Seizure frequencies up to 40 per month leave patients without any significant social life. Eighty percent of the patients with primary epilepsy will respond to pharmacologic treatment, however, according to the American Epilepsy foundation as many as 20% will not become completely seizure-free with antiepileptic medication alone [3, 20–22]. With a prevalence between 0.5 and 1.0 percent for epileptic disorders, a large number of patients with pharmacoresistant epilepsy can be anticipated in Germany, Austria and Switzerland. These patients are primarily candidates for epilepsy surgery or other treatment alternatives. Following temporal lobe resection (TLR) between 50 and 70% will experience freedom from seizures, another 20–30% will at least respond with a reduction in seizure frequency [3, 22]. Possible surgical risks, however, including neuropsychological deficits, have to be considered after TLR [17].

In patients with pharmacoresistant epilepsy and unsuccessful surgery or contraindications against TLR, fractionated stereotactic radiotherapy (SRT) remains a possible treatment option. It was the primary goal of this phase I/II trial to achieve permanent symptom control or to reduce seizure frequency and severity. At the same time SRT is characterized by potential advantages as it is a non-invasive technique without surgical risk. Late treatment associated toxicity can be minimized by the fractionated approach [1, 9, 24].

Patients and Methods

Inclusion Criteria

Patients aged between 18 and 65 years with pharmacoresistant temporal lobe epilepsy with unilateral focus were included in this study. Surgical options had to be fully exploited prior to trial entry. Exclusion criteria were epileptic foci without clear localisation, immunodeficiency syndrome with elevated radiosensitivity and pregnancy. Study endpoints were quantification of seizure frequency, in-

Table 1. *Patient Characteristics*

Pat no.	Localisation of epileptogenic focus	Gender	Age	Anticonvulsive medication	95%-Isodose (cm^3)	Dose (Gy)
01	Temporomesial l	f	24	4	10	21
02	Temporal-neocortical l	f	25	1	52	21
03	Temporomesial r	m	44	1	51	30
04	Temporomesial l	f	56	1	65	21
05	Occipital l	m	17	3	230	21
06	Temporodorsal l	m	37	2	126	28
07	Temporal-neocortical r	f	38	2	69	22.5
08	Temporomesial l	f	46	1	96	21
09	Temporomesial l	m	61	2	49	29
10	Parietal r	m	38	3	61	21
11	Frontodorsal r	f	26	4	160	29
12	Temporomesial l	m	28	2	12	30

m Male, *f* female.

tensity and duration as well as neuropsychological parameters. An interim analysis after treatment of six patients should specifically assess safety of this procedure.

Patients

A total of 7 female (58%) and 5 male patients (42%) were included being between 18 and 61 years old. Table 1 gives an overview on patients' characteristics. Three patients had prior unsuccessful TLR, all other patients were considered inoperable with epileptic foci located in or next to eloquent areas. Some patients were considered inoperable due to poor neuropsychologic baseline results. Written consent was obtained from all patients prior to trial entry, and the study protocol had been approved by the local ethics committee. Follow-up intervals were compatible with those following epilepsy surgery, i.e. 3, 6, 12, 24 months after SRT.

Design of Treatment Volume

Treatment volume of SRT was basically identical to the theoretical extent of surgical resection in temporal lobe epilepsy. Baseline diagnostic procedures for delineation of the epileptogenic area included medical history, neurologic examination, Video-EEG monitoring according to the international 10/20 system (Siemens-Mingograf EEG21), and invasive recordings via sphenoidal electrodes in two patients. In addition to MRI imaging (Siemens Magnetom, 1.5 Tesla), and MEG [23] ictual and interictual single photon emission computed tomography (SPECT) was performed to identify areas with low perfusion. Positron emission tomography (PET) using 18-fluorodeoxyglucose (^{18}FDG) was used in several cases to characterize hypometabolic foci in patients with unclear findings otherwise. The planning target volume was determined on an individual basis taking into account all available imaging data including morphological and functional measurements.

Radiotherapy

Fractionated SRT was delivered using 6 MV photons of a linear accelerator. Patients were immobilized in a face mask system [1]. For treatment planning, the PINNACLE^3 (ADAC Laboratories, Milpitas, CA., USA) planning system was utilised. The epileptogenic area was entirely covered by the 90–95% isodose line with a 5 mm safety margin (see Fig. 1).

The first six patients were irradiated with single fractions of 300 cGy up to a total dose of 2100 cGy. After a planned interim analysis which revealed a relatively promising reduction in seizure frequency but conflicting neuropsychological findings, it was decided to reduce the single fraction size to 200 cGy with a total dose of 3000 cGy. Mean duration of treatment as an inpatient was 13.5 days (range 9–24 days) with a mean of 9.6 treatment days (range 7–15 days). Table 1 gives an overview on the treatment parameters.

Neuropsychological Testing

All patients had intensive neuropsychological tests before SRT and in 3-month intervals thereafter. All methods have been previously described by Pauli *et al.* (1999).

Results

All patients experienced a marked reduction in seizure frequency, which reached a mean value of 46% over the first 18 months of follow-up. Taking into account only the seizure frequency over a 3 month period after a minimum follow-up of 1.5 years, the mean reduction was 37%. Table 2 gives mean quaterly seizure frequencies for all 11 evaluable patients during the first 18 months follow-up. The mean absolute value was reduced from 11.75 seizures to 7.45 seizures per month. Final results are shown in Table 3 displaying mean seizure frequencies prior to SRT and those experienced with a minimum follow-up of 1.5 years. Figure 2 gives seizure frequencies comparing those prior to RT with the mean values during follow-up.

The effects of SRT became also evident in terms of seizure quality. Among all 11 patients the duration of seizures was reduced in 5 patients (46%), intensity of seizures as reported by patients and relatives dimin-

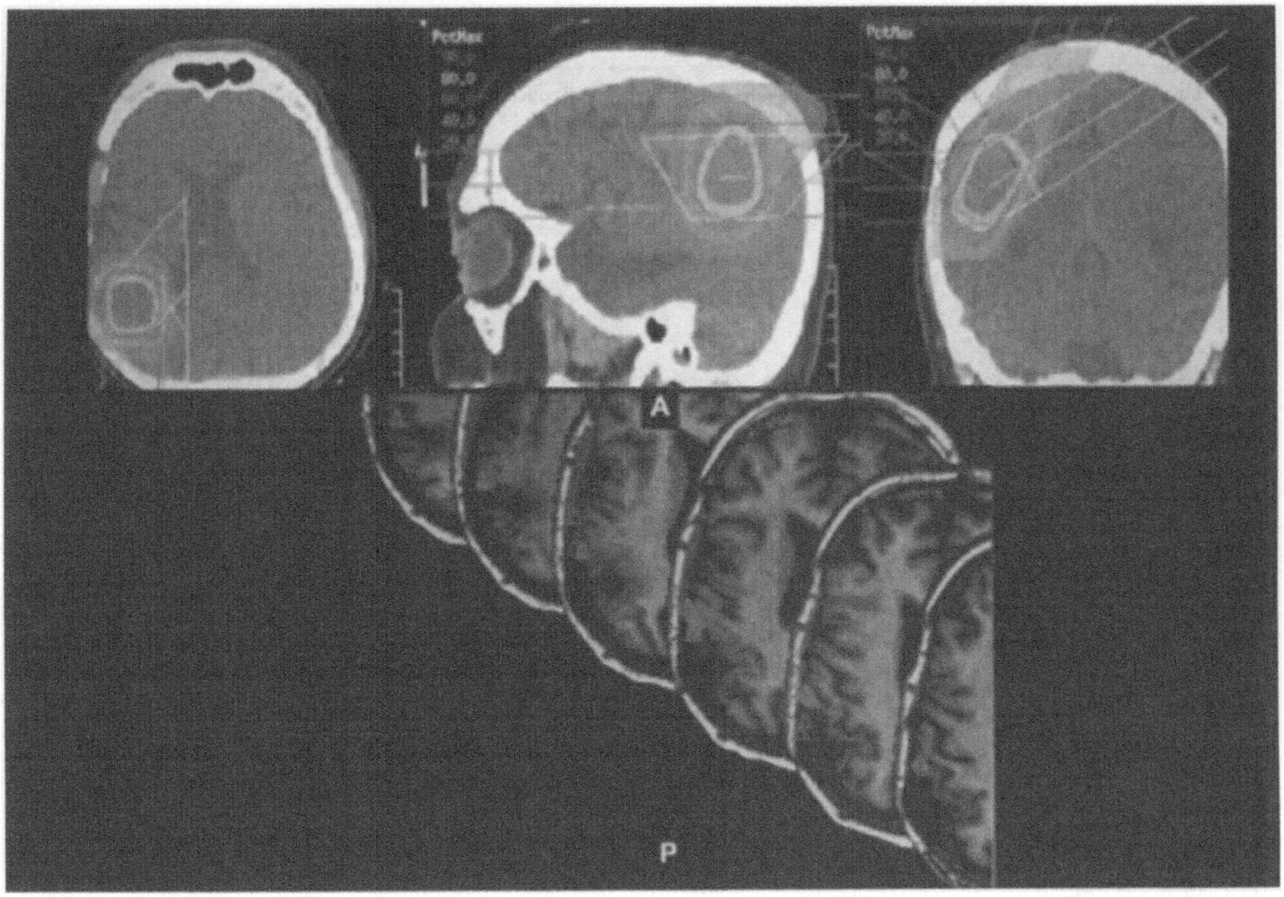

Fig. 1. Dose distribution in axial, sagittal frontal and reconstruction in a patient with temporal lobe epilepsy. 95% isodose line completely covers abnormal MEG signals

Table 2. *Seizure Frequency: Course During Follow-up. Numbers are Expressed as Mean Values of 3 Consecutive Months*

Seizure frequency							
Patient	Before RT	+3 Months	+6 Months	+9 Months	+12 Months	+15 Months	+18 Months
01	32.75	23.67	24.67	22	18.33	25.33	23.33
02	6	4	1.67	4	5.33	4	5
03	11	6.3	5.3	2.7	4.3	4.3	5.3
04	8	1	4	6	7.3	7	7.3
05	7	6.7	6.7	5.7	5.7	6	6.3
06	15	4.5	4.5	4.5	4.5	4.5	4.5
07	19.5	16	12.3	17.7	18	13	14.3
08	7	4	4	3.7	4.7	4.3	4.6
09	7.5	5	6	6.3	5.3	4.3	5.7
10	3	0	0	0	0.3	0	0.7
11	12.5	9.7	6.3	5.3	6	7	5.7
Median	11.75	7.35	6.86	7.08	7.25	7.22	7.52

RT Radiotherapy.

ished in 7 patients (64%). Finally patients received a questionnaire upon the overall results of the treatment. Six patients (60%) had the impression of a successful treatment, one patient was undecided and 3 patients reported no clinical benefit.

A majority of the patients tolerated SRT extremely well with no side effects in 5 patients. During treatment, 2 patients experienced seizures, 3 patients suffered from local transient alopecia, another 3 patients complained of headache or transient nausea. Only in

Table 3. *Seizure Frequency Comparing Values Before RT with Mean Number During 18 Months Follow-up and Mean Number at 18 Months after RT*

Patient no.	Number of seizures before RT	Seizures after RT (Mean during 18 mos)	Reduction (%)	Seizures after RT (Mean at 18 mos)	Reduction (%)
01	32.75	22.9	−30.08	23.33	−28.76
02	6	3.4	−43.33	5	−16.67
03	11	4.94	−55.05	5.3	−51.81
04	8	5.4	−32.50	7.3	−8.75
05	7	4	−42.86	6.3	−10
06	15	4.5	−70.0	4.5	−70
07	19.5	15	−23.08	14.3	−26.67
08	7	4.4	−37.14	4.6	−34.29
09	7.5	5.3	−29.33	5.7	−24
10	3	0.17	−94.33	0.7	−76.67
11	12.5	6.6	−47.20	5.7	−54.4
Median	11.75	6.96	−45.9%	7.52	−36.55%

RT Radiotherapy.

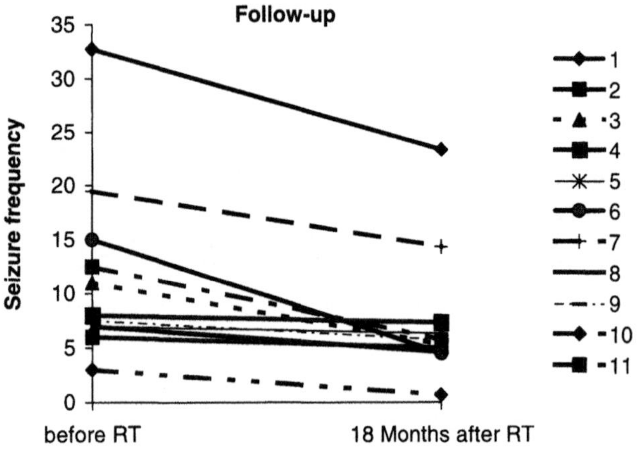

Fig. 2. Seizure frequency comparing mean monthly seizures prior to RT with outcome 18 months thereafter for all evaluable 11 patients

Table 4. *Neuropsychological Results Comparing Findings Prior to Stereotactic Radiotherapy with those at 18 Month Follow-up*

Patient no.	Memory functions after SRT	Verbal functions after SRT
01	−1 SD	−2 SD
02	±0	±0
03	−1 SD	±0
04	−1,5 SD	±0
05	No Test (Oligophrenia)	
06	>−2 SD	−1 SD
07	±0	±0
08	ca. −2 SD	−2 SD
09	−1,5 SD	±0
10	No Test (Compliance)	
11	±0	±0

SD Standard deviation.

one patient treatment was interrupted for 1 day secondary to severe nausea, which was then managed with steroids for several days.

Table 4 gives the results of neuropsychological evaluation prior to SRT and during follow-up. Results are displayed as standard deviations (SD) from age adjusted mean values. The left column represents the findings for memory function the right one for language performance. As for memory functions three patients had no changes, a deviation of up to − 1.5 SD was noted in 4 patients (45%), in two patients an increasing memory deficit of more than 2 SD was diagnosed. In terms of verbal functional parameters, six of nine evaluable patients (67%) had no significant changes, the remainder a reduction between 1 and 2 SD.

Discussion

It has been the aim of this pilot study to evaluate safety and long-term efficacy of SRT for treatment of a distinct subgroup of patients with pharmacoresistant temporal lobe epilepsy who were no candidates for TLR. All patients experienced a clinical benefit up to a minimum follow-up time of 18 months with a mean reduction in seizure frequency of 46%. Intensity of seizures was reduced in 64% and the duration in 46% of the patients. Following SRT, one third of the patients had a reduction in seizure frequency of more than 50%, another third between 30 and 50%, and the remaining group of up to 30%. This is superior to the results achieved after vagal nerve stimulation [5, 20] where one third of the patients did not have any clinical benefit.

Another approach has been the use of stereotactic radiosurgery (SRS) with one large single dose being applied to a very small treatment volume [2, 18, 19]. Gamma-knife SRS was applied in a series of patients with clearly diagnosed temporally located epileptic foci as an alternative to open surgery [18]. With this approach not all patients, however, became seizure-free and eventually TLR was necessary [12]. Also Barcia *et al.*. reported on 2/11 patients who failed after radiosurgery using 2×10 Gy. Major limitation of this approach seems to be that for exact delineation of the focus for later SRS invasive recordings are mandatory. In addition, possible long-term toxicity including brain necrosis may be associated with SRS [15]. Another experimental approach introduced into discussion recently is the repetitive transcranial magnetic stimulation. Positive effects were only seen up to a time interval between 6 and 8 weeks following treatment, however, two out of nine patients experienced no significant clinical benefit at all [25].

Exact localisation of the epileptogenic focus by non-invasive methods remains the major prerequisite for SRT. Besides EEG recordings we have been using all other available imaging tools including MRI, MEG, SPECT and PET to delineate the region of seizure generation as exactly as possible, particularly with the intention to reduce late radiation damage to normal brain tissue. Given the large number of contraindications against epilepsy surgery in patients within this pilot study, invasive recordings were only performed in selected cases. Future developments will also focus on chemical shift spectroscopy to identify regions with lower concentrations of N-acetyl aspartate [4, 8, 10, 16].

It has been emphasized that the patient population in this study mainly consisted of severe treatment resistant cases with a-priori reduced neuropsychologic performance. A continuous deterioration of these parameters even without surgery or SRT may be suspected during longer follow-up. Epileptic seizures per se as well as the long-term use of antiepileptic medications are presumably associated with adverse neuropsychological effects [14]. In addition, comorbidity like depression and day to day difference in performance may also have significant influence on neuropsychological test results. Following epilepsy surgery one patient in this study experienced severe memory deficits between 4 and 5 SD below the age adjusted mean values, which was more pronounced than those deficits seen after SRT. According to literature data standard temporal lobe resection of the dominant hemisphere has been associated with significant persisting neuropsychological deficits [17].

In conclusion, SRT is a non-invasive, safe and effective treatment for patients with pharmacoresistant temporal lobe epilepsy. Further studies in larger patient populations will specifically evaluate the role of optimal focus identification by newer imaging tools and will also include refinements in SRT techniques and assessment of a possible dose response relationship.

References

1. Alheit H, Dornfeld S, Dawel M, Alheit M, Henzel B, Steckler K, Blank H, Geyer P (2001) Patient position reproducibility in fractionated stereotactically guided conformal radiotherapy using the BrainLab mask system. Strahlenther Onkol 177: 264–268
2. Barcia JA, Barcia-Salorio JL, Lopez-Gomez L, Hernandez G (1994) Stereotactic radiosurgery may be effective in the treatment of idiopathic epilepsy: report on the methods and results in a series of eleven cases. Stereotact Funct Neurosurg 63: 271–279
3. Brodie MJ, French JA (2000) Management of epilepsy in adolescents and adults. Lancet 356: 323–329
4. Cendes F, Andermann F, Preul MC *et al* (1994) Lateralization of temporal lobe epilepsy based on regional metabolite abnormalities in proton magnetic resonance spectroscopic images. Ann Neurol 35: 211–216
5. Chadwick D (2001) Vagal-nerve stimulation for epilepsy. Lancet 357: 1726–1727
6. Eberhardt KE, Stefan H, Buchfelder M, Pauli E, Hopp P, Huk W, Tomandl BF (2000) The significance of bilateral CSI changes for the postoperative outcome in temporal lobe epilepsy. J Comput Assist Tomogr 24: 919–926
7. Eberhardt KE, Stefan H, Grabenbauer GG, Schäfer I, Tomandl B, Huk WJ, Kreisler P, Käferlein M (1999) Chemical shift imaging spectroscopy findings before and after stereotactic radiotherapy in temporal lobe epilepsy. Adv Neurol 81: 339–345
8. Gadian DC, Connelly A, Duncan JS *et al* (1994) ^{1}H magnetic resonance spectroscopy in the investigation of intractable epilepsy. Acta Neurol Scand 152: 116–121
9. Grabenbauer GG, Rödel C, Paulus W, Ganslandt O, Schuchardt U, Buchfelder M, Schrell U, Fahlbusch R, Huk WJ, Sauer R (2000) Supratentorial low-grade glioma: results and prognostic factors following postoperative radiotherapy. Strahlenther Onkol 176: 259–264
10. Hetherington H, Kuzniecky R, Pan J *et al* (1995) Proton nuclear magnetic resonance spectroscopic imaging of human temporal lobe epilepsy at 4.1 T. Ann Neurol 38: 396–404
11. Jouvenceau A, Eunson LH, Spauschus A, Ramesh V, Zuberi SM, Kullmann DM, Hanna MG (2001) Human epilepsy associated with dysfunction of the brain P/Q-type calcium channel. Lancet 358: 801–807
12. Kawai K, Suzuki I, Kurita H, Shin M, Arai N, Kirino T (2001) Failure of low-dose radiosurgery to control temporal lobe epilepsy. J Neurosurg 95: 883–887
13. Knowlton RC, Laxer KD, Ende G *et al* (1997) Presurgical multimodality neuroimaging in electroencephalographic lateralized temporal lobe epilepsy. Ann Neurol 42: 829–837

14. Kwan P, Brodie MJ (2001) Neuropsychological effects of epilepsy and antiepileptic drugs. Lancet 357: 216–222
15. Mitsumori M, Shrieve DC, Alexander E *et al* (1998) Initial clinical results of linac based stereotactic radiosurgery and stereotactic radiotherapy for pituitary adenomas. Int J Radiat Oncol Biol Phys 42: 573–580
16. Ng TC, Comair YG, Xue M *et al* (1993) Temporal lobe epilepsy: presurgical localization with proton chemical shift imaging. Radiology 193: 465–472
17. Pauli E, Pickel S, Schulemann H, Buchfelder M, Stefan H (1999) Neuropsychologic findings depending on the type of the resection in temporal lobe epilepsy. Adv Neurol 81: 371–377
18. Regis J, Bartolomei F, Rey M, Hayashi M, Chauvel P, Peragut JC (2000) Gamma knife surgery for mesial temporal lobe epilepsy. J Neurosurg 93 [Suppl] 3: 141–146
19. Regis J, Bartolomei F, Rey M, Genton P, Dravet C, Semah F, Gastaut JL, Chauvel P, Peragut JC (1999) Gamma knife surgery for mesial temporal lobe epilepsy. Epilepsia 40: 1551–1556
20. Scherrmann J, Hoppe C (2001) Vagusnerv-Stimulation. Dt Ärzteblatt 98: 990–992
21. Stefan H, Hummel C, Grabenbauer GG, Müller RG, Robeck S, Hofmann W, Buchfelder M (1998) Successful treatment of focal epilepsy be fractionated stereotactic radiotherapy. Eur Neurol 39: 248–250
22. Stefan H (1998) Epilepsietherapie. Dt Ärztebl 96: 3128–3137
23. Stefan H, Hummel C, Hopfengärtner R, Pauli E, Tilz C, Ganslandt O, Kober H, Moler A, Buchfelder M (2000) Magnetoencephalography in extratemporal epilepsy. J Clin Neurophysiol 17: 190–200
24. Sweeney RA, Bale R, Auberger T, Vogele M, Förster S, Nevinny-Stickel M, Lukas P (2001) A simple and non-invasive vacuum mouthpiece-based head fixation system for high-precision radiotherapy. Strahlenther Onkol 177: 43–47
25. Tergau F, Naumann U, Paulus W, Steinhoff BJ (1999) Low-frequency repetitive transcranial magnetic stimulation improves intractable epilepsy. Lancet 353: 2209

Correspondence: G. G. Grabenbauer, M.D., Department of Radiation Therapy, Universitätsstraße 27, 91054 Erlangen, Germany.

Acta Neurochir (2002) [Suppl] 84: 71–76

Preservation of Cranial Nerve Function Following Gamma Knife Radiosurgery for Benign Skull Base Meningiomas: Experience in 121 Patients with Follow-up of 5 to 9.8 Years

S. Eustacchio, M. Trummer, I. Fuchs, O. Schröttner, B. Sutter, and **G. Pendl**

Department of Neurosurgery, Karl-Franzens University, Graz, Austria

Summary

Introduction. Microsurgical excision with preservation of juxtaposed neurovascular structures is considered the treatment of choice for skull base meningiomas, but there exists a great controversy regarding surgical resectability, potential risk for subsequent postoperative Cranial Nerve Deficit (CND) and the role of adjuvant or adjunctive treatment options. In this study we evaluated the effect of Gamma Knife Radiosurgery (GKRS) in 121 patients with benign basal meningiomas after a follow-up of 5 to 9.8 years.

Methods. Sixty patients had undergone open resections prior to radiosurgical treatment and 61 patients were treated by GKRS alone. Tumour volumes of 0.5 to 89.9 ccm (median 6.8 ccm) received a median marginal dose of 13 Gy (range 7–25 Gy) at the covering 25% to 80% isodose volume curves (median 45%).

Results. Neuroradiological controls demonstrated decreased tumour size in 73 patients (60.3%), stable meningioma volume in 47 cases (38.9%) and tumour enlargement in one patient (0.8%). Clinically, 54 patients (44.6%) improved and 61 cases (50.4%) remained unchanged. Four patients (3.3%) showed temporary and two patients (1.7%) permanent neurological deterioration (unrelated to tumour or treatment in one patient). Two patients (1.7%) developed radiation induced new or aggravated pre-existent CND (1 transient, 1 permanent) and two patients (1.7%) required further surgical resection.

Conclusion. In our long-term experience, GKRS proved to be an attractive additional and save alternative primary treatment option in selected patients with basal meningiomas. The tumour control rate of 98.3% associated with excellent clinical outcome and low incidence for treatment related CND (1.7%) compares favourably with the reported microsurgical series.

Keywords: Gamma Knife; radiosurgery; skull base; meningioma.

Introduction

Total removal of the meningioma with resection or coagulation of the whole area of dural involvement or attachment and conservation of adjacent functional structures is considered the treatment of first choice [4, 7, 10, 24, 25, 29, 36, 38]. Due to the anatomic complexity of the skull base the complete resection or attempted total excision of these tumours may be associated with considerable postoperative Cranial Nerve Deficit (CND) and occasional mortality [2, 5, 7–10, 15, 33–37, 42]. Especially in patients in poor clinical condition is the extent of surgical resection more likely limited to partial resection than to achieve complete excision in order to minimize additional surgically induced morbidity [4, 7].

The short to interim experience with Gamma Knife Radiosurgery (GKRS) for treatment of benign skull base meningiomas has given excellent results concerning growth control, clinical outcome and complication rate [1, 11, 18, 23, 27, 30, 31, 31, 39]. Thus the management of basal meningiomas frequently requires weighing the potential risks of severe or life threatening postoperative sequelae following aggressive surgical procedures against the potential benefits offered by partial resection and subsequent radiosurgical treatment or GKRS alone [1, 2, 3, 8–10, 15, 32, 39]. As only a few publications report on long-term results after radiosurgical treatment of basal meningiomas [19, 20] we analysed the outcome – with special regard to the cranial nerve function – of our patients who received radiosurgical treatment for partially removed, recurrent, progressively growing residual or newly diagnosed skull base meningiomas with 5- to 9.8-year follow-up to provide further data for the ongoing debate.

Material and Methods

Between April 1992 and January 1997, 121 patients with benign skull base meningiomas underwent radiosurgery with the Leksell

Table 1. *Distribution of Pre- and Postradiosurgical Cranial Nerve Deficits (CND) in 121 Patients with Skull Base Meningiomas*

Deficit of cranial nerve	At time of GKRS no. of patients (%)	Subsided after GKRS no. of patients (%)	Improved after GKRS no. of patients (%)	Unchanged after GKRS no. of patients (%)	Worsened after GKRS no. of patients (%)
I	4 (3.3)			4 (3.3)	
II	44 (36.4)	5 (4.1)	7 (5.8)	30 (24.8)	2* (1.7)
III	25 (20.6)	4 (3.3)	9 (7.4)	12 (9.9)	
IV	7 (5.8)	2 (1.7)		5 (4.1)	
V	26 (21.5)	3 (2.5)	13 (10.7)	10 (8.3)	1** (0.8)
VI	16 (13.2)	6 (4.9)	3 (2.5)	7 (5.8)	
VII	8 (6.6)	3 (2.5)	1 (0.8)	4 (3.3)	
VIII	10 (8.3)			10 (8.3)	
IX+X	4 (3.3)			4 (3.3)	
XI	1 (0.8)			1 (0.8)	
XII	2 (1.7)		1 (0.8)	1 (0.8)	

* Including transient deterioration of pre-existent visual field defect in one patient with tumour progression.
** Transient new onset of CND following GKRS.

Table 2. *Specific Tumour Location in 121 Patients with Benign Basal Meningiomas*

Location	No. of tumours
Cavernous sinus	45
Petroclival	26
Sphenoid wing	18
Cerebellopontine angle	11
Olfactory groove	8
Orbital	7
Intra- and suprasellar	3
Ventral foramen magnum	3
Total	121

Gamma Knife model B at the Department of Neurosurgery, Karl-Franzens University of Graz. The median age of the 23 male and 98 female patients was 56 years (range 10 to 78 years). Sixty patients had undergone between 1 and 4 microsurgical operations 0.2–182.6 months (median 3.9 months) prior to GKRS. In 4 cases with very large meningiomas (19 to 89.9 ccm), we performed staged radiosurgical procedures with 4.6–6.2 month intervals between partial volume treatments (median 6 months) [32]. For personal reasons one of these patients with a large petroclival meningioma decided to receive the third radiosurgical treatment after an interval of 83.8 months. Sixty-one patients with the typical characteristics of benign meningiomas on computerized tomography (CT) and/or magnetic resonance imaging (MRI) had primary GKRS due to medical infirmity, advanced age or refusal to undergo open surgery. The distribution of presenting CND at the time of GKRS and the locations of the skull base meningiomas are detailed in tables 1 and 2, respectively.

All patients but a 10 year-old male had the stereotactic frame fixed under local anaesthesia. High-resolution contrast-enhanced CT or gadolinium-enhanced MRI were performed to define tumour localization and its relation to juxtaposed structures. Caliber measurements in three separate dimensions were made before and after GKRS and tumour enlargement or regression was defined as a change of ± 2 mm. Volumetry was calculated at the time of GKRS but not available for all cases in the follow-up because several imaging studies were performed at the local radiologist. With the aid of the Kula or GammaPlan software multiple isocenter computer dose planning was completed to create radiation fields that conformed precisely to the often irregular shape of the meningioma (median number of isocenters 5, range 1–14 isocenters). Dose selection, guided by dose-volume analysis of prior radiosurgical series [14, 21, 38] and our prior experience in the management of meningiomas [22, 30, 31] was tailored to each case on the basis of specific tumour volume, location and the projected radiobiological risk of adjacent neural structures. The median tumour volume was 6.8 ccm (range 0.5–89.9 ccm). The tumour borders were covered by isodose lines ranging from 25–80% (median 45%). In the early years marginal doses up to 25 Gy were delivered to the meningioma surface but were decreased later to an average of 13 Gy (range 7–25 Gy). Maximum doses delivered to the tumour center ranged from 15 to 56.6 Gy (median 30 Gy). All patients were discharged the day after GKRS.

Clinical and neuroradiological follow-up examinations were performed at 6 months, at 1-year intervals for the first five years, and if the tumour volume remained stable or decreased, the interval was extended to 2 years thereafter.

Results

During the observation period of 60 to 117 months (median 82 months) the follow-up scans demonstrated a reduction in tumour size in 73 patients (60.3%) and stable tumour volume in 47 cases (38.9%). In the remaining patient (0.8%) the cavernous sinus meningioma resumed growing 77 months after combined surgical and radiosurgical treatment and the patient underwent further microsurgical resection. Central loss of contrast enhancement indicating marked tumour necrosis was found in the follow-up studies of 32 patients (26.4%). Massive peritumoural oedema developed in two patients (1.7%) 3.6 and 6 months after secondary GKRS of cavernous sinus meningiomas, but completely resolved after oral application of dexamethasone.

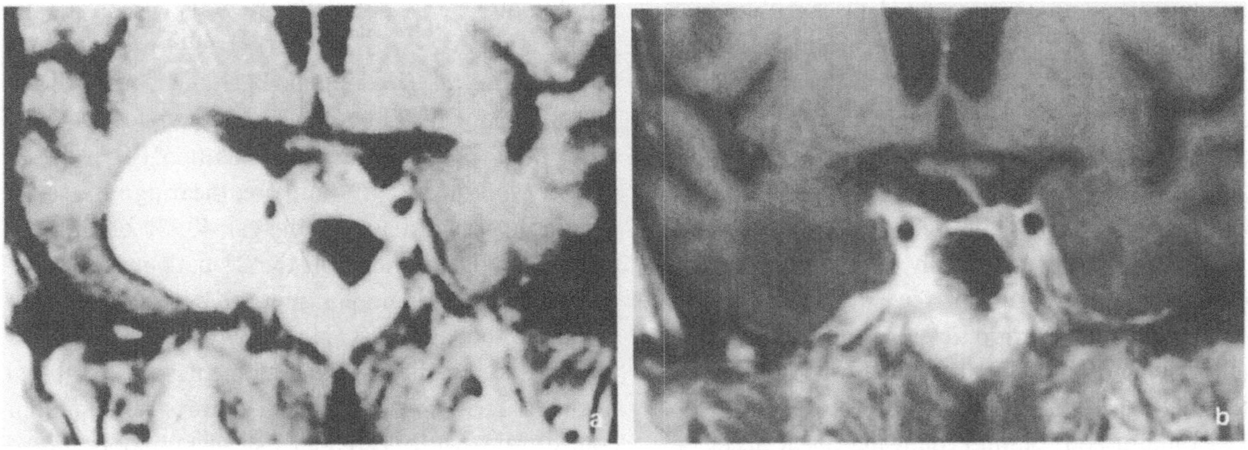

Fig. 1. (a) T1-weighted gadolinium-enhanced cranial MRI (coronal view) displaying a right-sided cavernous sinus meningioma in a 64-year-old patient with a 2 month history of diplopia due to ipsilateral abducent nerve palsy. As the patient refused to undergo microsurgical treatment primary GKRS was performed applying a marginal dose of 12 Gy at the enveloping 30% isodose line. During the course of the following two years a remarkable tumour shrinkage was noted on the imaging controls. (b) Latest MRI, obtained 95 months after GKRS, demonstrating unchanged reduced tumour size. Clinically, the abducent nerve palsy subsided 1 year after GKRS and the patient's neurological status has turned to normal

Clinical evaluation showed improved preradiosurgical deficits in 54 patients (44.6%), thirteen of which (10.7%) were found with normal neurological status. The neurological disorders remained unchanged in 61 patients (50.4%), while 4 cases (3.3%) experienced transient and two patients (1.7%) permanent clinical deterioration. In the 91 patients suffering from impaired function of one or more cranial nerves prior to GKRS CND completely resolved in 11 patients (12.1%), improved in 32 patients (35.2%) and remained stable in 45 patients (49.4%). Three of these 91 patients (3.3%) developed new (1 transient) or worsened pre-existent (1 temporary, 1 persistent) CND. The distribution of pre- and postradiosurgical CND is listed in Table 1. The temporary visual disturbances of the only patient with an enlarged meningioma resolved completely after further resection. The disappearance of radiation induced oedema in two patients was associated with normalization of their clinical disorders (increased seizure activity and aggravation of headache). Twelve months after secondary GKRS the fourth patient with passing clinical deterioration experienced new onset of trigeminal neuralgia. On follow-up imaging the tumour volume was unchanged and the trigeminal neuralgia subsided within the following weeks. Permanent worsening was not related to GKRS or tumour but caused by stroke in one patient. The persistent deterioration of visual field defect occurring 5.5 months after combined treatment of a cavernous sinus meningioma in another patient with stable tumour size showed only partial improvement following repeated microsurgery and was therefore presumed to be the second radiation-induced CND. Two patients with reduced tumour volume and ameliorated neurological status died 96 and 71 months after GKRS from unrelated disease (lymphoblastic cancer and pneumonia) at the age of 72 and 82 years, respectively.

Discussion

Complete removal of basal meningiomas with resection or coagulation of the dural base is considered the treatment of choice, but due to their close proximity to important neurovascular structures partial resection was performed in 12.5 to 40% of the microsurgically treated patients to reduce the risk for postoperative neurological impairment [2, 5, 7–10, 15, 33–37, 42]. Nevertheless, the most important surgical morbidity has been new or aggravated pre-existent CND, resolving during the postoperative course in 20 to 44% but persisting in 16 to 56% of the patients [2, 5, 7, 8, 10, 15, 33, 34, 36, 37]. Mortality following microsurgery has been reported to range between 0 and 9% (average mortality 3.6%) [2, 5, 7–10, 15, 33–37, 42]. The recurrence rate of basal meningiomas increases steeply with the duration of the follow-up period and seems to be influenced by extent of microsurgical resection, tumour site and specific histopathological features, as well [2, 3, 5, 7–10, 15, 24, 25, 33–37, 42]. Furthermore, complete removal may not be feasible or advisable in patients with advanced age, poor clinical condition, associated disease, high-risk tumour location and residual or recurrent skull base meningiomas, so that less invasive treatment strategies should be taken into account for the therapeutic management of these patients [1, 2, 7, 10, 20, 21, 27, 30, 31, 35, 38–40].

Conventional irradiation reduced the recurrence rates in unresectable or partially excised benign meningiomas, but up to 19% of the patients died from uncontrollable tumour progression, and treatment related optic neuropathy occurred in 1.6 to 2.5% of the patients [4, 16, 17, 24, 29, 40].

The tumour control rates following linear accelerator-based radiosurgery for benign basal meningiomas varied between 93.3 and 98%. The treatment related mortality rate ranged from 0 to 6.7%. A transient CND was observed in 1.8 to 18.2% of the Linac series, and 3.6 to 6.7 % of the patients experienced permanent worsening of cranial nerve function [6, 12, 44].

Short- to mid-term tumour control rates of 92 to 100% have been achieved after GKRS for skull base meningiomas with 0 to 18.2% of the patients developing transient and 0 to 8.8% suffering from permanent cranial nerve palsies. To date, no Gamma Knife series reported a treatment related death [1, 11, 18, 23, 26, 27, 30–32, 39]. Unlike surgical resection, the aim of which is complete tumour removal, the goal of GKRS is long-term prevention of tumour growth with maintenance of neurological function so that longer observation periods are necessary to define the role of GKRS for basal meningiomas [1, 9, 20, 21, 28, 38, 39].

In the present Gamma Knife series with 5 to almost 10 years follow-up further progression of skull base meningiomas could be stopped in 98.3%. The temporary worsened visual acuity in the only patient with a progressive cavernous sinus meningioma completely resolved after reoperation and was therefore a direct result from tumour compression and not caused by radiation injury. The permanently deteriorated vision in one patient (0.8%) and transient new trigeminal neuralgia in another patient (0.8%) accounted for an 1.7% incidence of radiation induced CND following GKRS. At 5 to 10 years follow-up Kondziolka *et al.* [20] observed tumour control in 93% of the 99 patients undergoing GKRS for meningioma treatment. Within 3 to 31 months after GKRS two patients (2%) experienced new deterioration of cranial nerve function (1 transient abducent nerve palsy, 1 persisting hemianopsia) and further deterioration of pre-existent CND was found in another two patients (1 permanent occulomotor nerve palsy, 1 temporary visual impairment). Following GKRS for benign meningiomas Kobayashi *et al.* [19] obtained tumour control in 48 out of 54 patients (88.9%) available for a follow-up of more than 5 years. Three patients (5.6%) developed new or worsened CND (impaired hearing in 2 cases, 1 reduced visual acuity), whereas 48.1% of the pre-existent CND improved in the 27 patients with cavernous sinus meningiomas after GKRS.

Within the last years, many Gamma Knife centers have reduced radiosurgical treatment doses for basal meningiomas achieving unchanged excellent tumour control rates with decreased risk of radiation related complications [18, 23, 28, 30, 31]. Currently, we assume that benign meningiomas should be treated with margin doses of 12 Gy, but the radiosensitivity of juxtaposed structures at risk sometimes necessitates to administer lower doses. The anterior visual pathways proved to be the most radiosensitive structures [11, 21, 22, 26, 38, 41]. According to our initial experience [22] they seemed to tolerate only doses of up to 10 Gy, while Morita *et al.* [26] found no radiation induced optic neuropathy, if doses of 10 to 16 Gy involved only short segments of the optic nerve, chiasm or tract. In contrast, other authors stated that even doses exceeding 8 or 9 Gy may cause visual impairment [11, 20, 21, 41]. In our current series the optic apparatus was at risk in 81 patients receiving doses between 3 to 12 Gy (median 8 Gy), but no part of the optic pathways was exposed to doses of more than 10 Gy in the only patient developing permanent optic neuropathy. The nerves controlling the ocular muscles appeared to be more radioresistent and were presumed to tolerate even doses beyond 20 Gy [11, 21, 22, 38], but Morita *et al.* found one patient with permanent new occulomotor nerve palsy after administration of 10 Gy to the cavernous sinus [26]. Nakaya *et al.* [28] reported occurrence of transient third cranial nerve injury in two patients following application of margin doses of 9.9 to 10 Gy and central doses of 20 to 25 Gy for meningioma treatment. Tishler *et al.* [41] cited one persistent worsened deficit of the third cranial nerve delivering a maximum dose of 40 Gy to the cavernous sinus. No Gamma Knife series documented radiation injury to the fourth cranial nerve, while abducent nerve palsy was observed in one patient following exposure of the cavernous sinus to a dose of 22 Gy [26]. The third, fourth and sixth cranial nerves in the 72 patients of our own series with these structures at risk received doses of 4 to 30 Gy (median 15 Gy), but no patient developed a radiogenic neuropathy after GKRS. The Pittsburgh group [21] related occurrence of 1 transient trigeminal hypaesthesia after delivering doses of 20–40 Gy to a petrous apex meningioma. In their other reports they did not detail specific information regarding treatment doses for the patients developing CND of the third (2 cases), fifth (2 cases) and sixth cranial nerve (4 cases) after GKRS of cavernous sinus, petroclival and intracranial meningiomas [11, 20, 21, 39]. Tishler *et al.* [41] noted radiation induced injury to the trigeminal nerve in two patients following Gamma Knife treatment with maximum cavernous sinus doses of 26 and 33.3 Gy, respectively. The observations of Morita *et al.*, who found increased incidence for trigeminal neuropathy following application of doses exceeding 19 Gy, did not reach statistical significance [26]. In our current series the fifth cranial nerves were exposed to doses ranging from 5 to 20 Gy (median 11 Gy) but new transient trigeminal neuralgia developed in one of our patients after receiving 12 to 17 Gy.

According to our experience in the radiosurgical treatment of vestibular schwannomas [43], maximum irradiation exposure of facial nerves was limited to 8–10 Gy (median 9.3 Gy) and marginal tumour dose to meningiomas of the cerebellopontine angle was not exceeding 12–14 Gy to avoid radiation damage to the eighth cranial nerve. Iwai *et al.* [18] observed deterioration of one facial nerve palsy following application of 12 Gy at the tumour borders, while the reports mentioning hearing deterioration after GKRS for meningioma treatment (3 cases) did not specify the treatment parameters for these patients [19, 39]. Results after GKRS of basal meningiomas demonstrated that the lower cranial nerves were not affected by currently recommended doses. Supported by our radiosurgical experience with glomus jugulare tumours [13] the ninth, tenth, eleventh and twelfth cranial nerves in our skull base meningioma series received maximum doses of 11.1–17.7 Gy (median 12 Gy) and no patient experienced exacerbation of pre-existent or development of new deficit of the lower cranial nerves.

Conclusion

The therapeutic management of basal meningiomas has to be tailored to each case according to age, general clinical condition, preoperative neurological deficit, specific tumour characteristics and patient preference. The rate of cranial nerve preservation after GKRS is superior to the results after microsurgery alone, but rapidly progressive neurological deficit, especially compression of the optic nerve or chiasm, is a clear indication for surgical resection. Nevertheless, the first priority is preservation of function so that in many cases it is advisable to remove a basal meningioma partially rather than to attempt radical resection since sacrification of cranial nerves or large blood vessels to remove remnants is not an acceptable risk nor a way to guarantee cure. Based on the well documented progression of incompletely resected meningiomas and the improved results following combined surgical-radiosurgical treatment, it seems wise to follow the partial removal of basal meningiomas with GKRS during the early postoperative interval (2–6 months). Patients with recurrent skull base meningiomas should rather be treated by GKRS than undergo repeated microsurgical resection. We recommend GKRS as safe and effective alternative primary treatment in elderly or medically infirm patients or if the risk of surgery in patients with meningiomas at critical location exceeds the potential benefit offered.

References

1. Aichholzer M, Bertalanffy A, Dietrich W, Roessler K, Pfisterer W, Ungersböck K, Heimberger K, Kitz K (2000) Gamma knife radiosurgery of skull base meningiomas. Acta Neurochir (Wien) 142: 647–653
2. Arnautović KI, Al-Mefty O, Husain M (2000) Ventral foramen magnum meningiomas. J Neurosurg 92 Spine 1: 71–80
3. Ayerbe J, Lobato RD, de la Cruz J, Alday R, Rivas JJ, Gómez PA, Cabrera A (1999) Risk factors predicting recurrence in patients operated on for intracranial meningioma. A multivariate analysis. Acta Neurochir (Wien) 141: 921–932
4. Barbaro NM, Gutin PH, Wilson CB, Sheline GE, Boldrey EB, Wara WM (1987) Radiation therapy in the treatment of partially resected meningiomas. Neurosurgery 20: 525–528
5. Bricolo AP, Turazzi S, Talacchi A, Cristofori L (1992) Microsurgical removal of petroclival meningiomas: a report of 33 patients. Neurosurgery 31: 813–828
6. Chang SD, Adler JR Jr (1997) Treatment of cranial base meningiomas with linear accelerator radiosurgery. Neurosurgery 41: 1019–1027
7. Couldwell WT, Fukushima T, Giannotta SL, Weiss MH (1996) Petroclival meningiomas: surgical experience in 109 cases. J Neurosurg 84: 20–28
8. Cusimano MD, Sekhar LN, Sen CN, Pomonis S, Wright DC, Biglan AW, Jannetta PJ (1995) The results of surgery for benign tumours of the cavernous sinus. Neurosurgery 37: 1–10
9. De Jesus O, Sekhar LN, Parikh HK, Wright DC, Wagner DP (1996) Long-term follow-up of patients with meningiomas involving the cavernous sinus: recurrence, progression, and quality of life. Neurosurgery 39: 915–920
10. DeMonte F, Smith HK, Al-Mefty O (1994) Outcome of aggressive removal of cavernous sinus meningiomas. J Neurosurg 81: 245–251
11. Duma CM, Lunsford LD, Kondziolka D, Harsh GF IV, Flickinger JC (1993) Stereotactic radiosurgery of cavernous sinus

meningiomas as an addition or alternative to microsurgery. Neurosurgery 32: 699–705
12. Engenhart R, Kimmig BN, Höver KH, Wowra B, Sturm V, van Kaick G, Wannenmacher M (1990) Stereotactic single high dose radiation therapy of benign intracranial meningiomas. Int J Radiat Oncol Biol Phys 19: 1021–1026
13. Eustacchio S, Leber K, Trummer M, Unger F, Pendl G (1999) Gamma knife radiosurgery for glomus jugulare tumours. Acta Neurochir (Wien) 141: 811–818
14. Flickinger JC (1989) An integrated logistic formula for prediction of complications from radiosurgery. Int J Radiat Oncol Biol Phys 17: 879–885
15. George B, Lot G, Boissonnet H (1997) Meningioma of the foramen magnum: a series of 40 cases. Surg Neurol 47: 371–379
16. Glaholm J, Bloom HJG, Crow JH (1990) The role of radiotherapy in the management of intracranial meningiomas: the Royal Marsden Hospital experience with 186 patients. Int J Radiat Oncol Biol Phys 18: 755–761
17. Goldsmith BJ, Wara WM, Wilson CB, Larson DA (1994) Postoperative irradiation for subtotally resected meningiomas. A retrospective analysis of 140 patients treated from 167 to 1990. J Neurosurg 80: 195–201
18. Iwai Y, Yamanaka K, Yasui T, Komiyama M, Nishikawa M, Nakajima H, Kishi H (1999) Gamma knife surgery for skull base meningiomas. The effectiveness of low-dose treatment. Surg Neurol 52: 40–45
19. Kobayashi T, Kida Y, Mori Y (2001) Long-term results of stereotactic gamma knife radiosurgery of meningiomas. Surg Neurol 55: 325–331
20. Kondziolka D, Levy EI, Niranjan A, Flickinger JC, Lunsford LD (1999) Long-term outcomes after meningioma radiosurgery: physician and patient perspectives. J Neurosurg 91: 44–50
21. Kondziolka D, Lunsford LD, Coffey RJ, Flickinger JC (1991) Stereotactic radiosurgery of meningiomas. J Neurosurg 74: 552–559
22. Leber KA, Berglöff J, Pendl G (1998) Dose-response tolerance of the visual pathways and cranial nerves of the cavernous sinus to stereotactic radiosurgery. J Neurosurg 88: 43–50
23. Liščák R, Šimonová G, Vymazal J, Janoušková L, Vladyka V (1999) Gamma knife radiosurgery of meningiomas in the cavernous sinus region. Acta Neurochir (Wien) 141: 473–480
24. Mathiesen T, Lindquist C, Kihlström L, Karlsson B (1996) Recurrence of cranial base meningiomas. Neurosurgery 39: 2–9
25. Mirimanoff RO, Dosoretz DE, Linggood RM, Ojemann RG, Martuza RL (1985) Meningioma: analysis of recurrence and progression following neurosurgical resection. J Neurosurg 62: 18–24
26. Morita A, Coffey RJ, Foote RL, Schiff D, Gorman D (1999) Risk of injury to cranial nerves after gamma knife radiosurgery for skull base meningiomas: experience in 88 patients. J Neurosurg 90: 42–49
27. Muthukumar N, Kondziolka D, Lunsford LD, Flickinger JC (1999) Stereotactic radiosurgery for anterior foramen magnum meningiomas. Surg Neurol 51: 268–273
28. Nakaya K, Hayashi M, Nakamura S, Atsuchi S, Sato H, Ochial T, Yamamoto M, Izawa M, Hori T, Takakura T (1999) Low-dose radiosurgery for meningiomas. Stereotact Funct Neurosurg 72 [Suppl] 1: 67–72
29. Nutting C, Brada M, Brazil L, Sibtain A, Saran F, Westbury C, Moore A, Thomas D, Traish D, Ashley S (1999) Radiotherapy in the treatment of benign meningioma of the skull base. J Neurosurg 90: 823–827
30. Pendl G, Schröttner O, Eustacchio S, Feichtinger K, Ganz J (1997) Stereotactic radiosurgery of skull base menigiomas. Minim Invas Neurosurg 40: 87–90
31. Pendl G, Schröttner O, Eustacchio S, Ganz JC, Feichtinger K (1998) Cavernous sinus meningioma – what is the strategy: upfront or adjuvant gamma knife surgery? Stereotact Funct Neurosurg 70 [Suppl] 1: 33–40
32. Pendl G, Unger F, Papaefthymiou G, Eustacchio S (2000) Staged radiosurgical treatment for large benign cerebral lesions (meningioma and AVM's). J Neurosurg 93 [Suppl] 3: 107–112
33. Samii M, Tatagiba M (1992) Experience with 36 surgical cases of petroclival meningiomas. Acta Neurochir (Wien) 118: 27–32
34. Samii M, Klekamp J, Carvalho G (1996) Surgical results for meningiomas of the craniocervical junction. Neurosurgery 39: 1086–1095
35. Samii M, Carvalho GA, Tatagiba M, Matthies C (1997) Surgical management of meningiomas originating in Meckel's cave. Neurosurgery 41: 767–775
36. Sekhar LN, Swamy NKS, Jaiswal V, Rubinstein E, Hirsch WE, Wright DC (1994) Surgical excision of meningiomas involving the clivus: preoperative and intraoperative features as predictors of postoperative functional deterioration. J Neurosurg 81: 860–868
37. Spallone A, Makhmudov UB, Mukhamedjanov DJ, Tcherekajev VA (1999) Petroclival meningioma. An attempt to define the role of skull base approaches in their surgical management. Surg Neurol 51: 412–420
38. Steiner L, Lindquist Ch, Steiner M (1991) Meningiomas and Gamma Knife radiosurgery. In: Al-Mefty O (ed) Meningiomas. Raven Press, New York, pp 263–272
39. Subach BR, Lunsford LD, Kondziolka D, Maitz AH, Flickinger JC (1998) Management of petroclival meningiomas by stereotactic radiosurgery. Neurosurgery 42: 437–445
40. Taylor BW Jr, Marcus RB Jr, Friedman WA, Ballinger WE Jr, Million RR (1988) The meningioma controversy: postoperative radiation therapy. Int J Radiat Oncol Biol Phys 15: 299–304
41. Tishler RB, Loeffler JS, Lunsford LD, Duma C, Alexander E III, Kooy HM, Flickinger JC (1993) Tolerance of cranial nerves of the cavernous sinus to radiosurgery. Int J Radiat Oncol Biol Phys 27: 215–221
42. Thomas NWM, King TT (1996) Meningiomas of the cerebellopontine angle. A report of 41 cases. Br J Neurosurg 10: 59–68
43. Unger F, Walch C, Haselsberger K, Papaefthymiou G, Trummer M, Eustacchio S, Pendl G (1999) Radiosurgery of vestibular schwannomas: a minimally invasive alternative to microsurgery. Acta Neurochir (Wien) 141: 1281–1286
44. Villavicencio AT, Black PM, Shrieve DC, Fallon MP, Alexander E, Loeffler JS (2001) Linac radiosurgery for skull base meningiomas. Acta Neurochir (Wien) 143: 1141–1152

Correspondence: Dr. Sandro Eustacchio, Department of Neurosurgery, Karl-Franzens University, Auenbruggerplatz 29, 8036 Graz, Austria.

Acta Neurochir (2002) [Suppl] 84: 77–83

Cranial Nerve Preservation after Radiosurgery of Vestibular Schwannomas

F. Unger[1], **C. Walch**[2], **O. Schröttner**[1], **S. Eustacchio**[1], **B. Sutter**[1], and **G. Pendl**[1]

[1] Department of Neurosurgery, Karl-Franzens University, Graz, Austria
[2] Department of Ear, Nose and Throat, Karl-Franzens University, Graz, Austria

Summary

Radiosurgery is a management approach used to treat patients with vestibular schwannomas. The goals are long-term tumour growth control, maintenance of cranial nerve function and prevention of new deficiencies. We sought to determine long-term outcomes measuring the potential benefits against the neurological risks of primary radiosurgery.

Gamma Knife radiosurgery was applied as a treatment modality for 289 patients with vestibular schwannomas from April 1992 to April 2002. The long-term results of 100 patients who underwent radiosurgery were evaluated. 60 patients received a primary treatment, 40 other cases presented with previously performed subtotal microsurgical resection or recurrence of disease (12–96 months, median 39). The median treatment volume was 3.4 ccm and the median dose to the tumour margin was 13 Gy. The median patient follow-up time was 76 months (range 60–120 months).

Four tumours progressed after primary radiosurgery. Tumour control rate was 96%. Useful hearing (Gardner-Robertson I/II) was preserved in 16 patients (55%). Clinical neurological improvement occured in 50%. Adverse effects comprised neurological symptoms (incomplete facial palsy) (House-Brackman II/III) in six cases (four recovered completely), mild transient trigeminal neuropathy in five cases, and morphological changes displaying rapid enlargement of preexisting macrocysts in two patients and tumour growth in two other patients. Microsurgical resection was performed in four cases (4%) and two patients underwent a shunting procedure because of hydrocephalus formation (2%).

In patients who had undergone previous microsurgery, no new cranial nerve deficit was observed.

Radiosurgery is an effective method for growth control of vestibular schwannomas and is associated with both a low mortality rate and a good quality of life. Accordingly, for the preservation of cranial nerve function radiosurgery is a useful method for the management of properly selected patients and is comparable to microsurgery.

Keywords: Acoustic neurinoma; cranial nerve preservation; radiosurgery; vestibular schwannoma.

Introduction

The outcome of surgical treatment of vestibular schwannomas has improved considerably regarding both facial nerve function and the preservation of residual hearing [16, 23, 24]. Nevertheless, open surgery in the cerebellopontine angle remains a challenging procedure with, at times unacceptably high risks. This applies particularly in cases with bilateral tumours or in patients with significant medical problems in particular, the elderly.

Taking into account the fact that neoplasms of this type grow slowly or even arrest, patients with small tumours have generally been advised to be observed or have been treated radiosurgically. Accordingly 40 cases of residual or recurrent tumours after previous microsurgical resection with long-term follow-up were added in this study to determine the efficacy of our technique.

Radiosurgery (RS) offers a minimally invasive method with a precise, mechanically directed, closed-skull destruction of an intracranial target. Unlike surgical resection, the goal of which is complete tumour removal, the goal of RS is long-term prevention of tumour growth with maintenance of neurological function.

As of April 30th 2002, 289 patients with vestibular schwannomas have been treated at our institution. This study analyses the long-term results with between 5 and 10 years after RS.

Materials and Methods

Patient Population

Between 1992 and 1996 Radiosurgery for vestibular schwannoma was performed on 140 patients at the University of Graz. The present series comprises 100 patients (58 males, 42 females) with a median age of 58 years (range 16–82 years) who underwent RS for vestibular schwannoma and were available with complete follow-up information. Resection had been previously performed in 40 patients over a

Table 1. *Characteristics of 60 Patients at the Time of Stereotactic Radiosurgery for Vestibular Schwannoma as Primary Treatment*

Characteristic	Value: primary RS	Adjunctive RS
1. Age (years)		
Median (range)	54 (16–81)	49 (16–79)
2. Volume (ccm)		
Median (range)	3.8 (0.02–27.22)	3.4 (0.2–23.09)
3. Hearing loss (no./%)*	50 patients/83%	40 pts./100%
Useful hearing	29 patients/48%	4 pts./10%
4. Facial nerve weakness (no./%)**	10 patients/17%	30 pts./75%
5. Tinnitus (no./%)	18 patients/30%	16 pts./40%
6. Imbalance (no./%)	18 patients/30%	14 pts./35%
7. Marginal dose (30–80%)		
Median (range)	12 Gy (9–18 Gy)	13 Gy (10–18 Gy)
8. Isocentres		
Median (range)	5 (1–12)	4 (1–11)

* Assessed with the Gardner-Robertson scale [7].
** Assessed with the House-Brackmann scale [10].

period of 12–96 months earlier (median 39) (in 74% in other neuro-/otosurgical institutions) and 12 of them represented with a recurrence of the disease which was radiographically documented after total resection. 31 patients had experienced a single surgical intervention, 6 were operated on twice and 3 other patients three or more times. In the majority of cases there was a small tumour residual adherent to either the facial nerve or the brain stem that was jugded to be impossible to resect without significant morbidity. Median follow-up was 76 months (range 60–120 months). 40 other patients were not available for complete follow-up. The clinical characteristics are shown in Table 1.

The majority of the tumours were located on the right side (57%), 11% were located intrameatally and 4 patients had bilateral tumours (neurofibromatosis II), only one side of which was treated radiosurgically. In more than one half of the patients (58%) maximum extrameatal tumour diameters ranged between 10 and 20 mm. Lesions measuring 20–30 mm were assessed in 24% of cases. Smaller (<10 mm diameter) and larger tumours (>30 mm diameter) accounted for 11% and 7%, of cases, respectively.

Postoperative Evaluation

Follow-up examinations performed at regular intervals of 6 months included MR-imaging and both neurological and otolaryngological examination. Contrast-enhanced imaging studies were used to define the tumour response and to identify hydrocephalus or other changes around the tumour. Before and after RS, separate caliber measurements (extracanicular and intracanicular) were made. Tumour enlargement or regression was defined as a change of ± 2 mm. Volumetry was calculated at the time of RS but was not available for all cases in the follow-up because several imaging studies were performed by peripheral radiologists.

Facial nerve function was assessed according to the grading system of House-Brackmann [10] (Table 3) whereas the functional evaluation of the 8th cranial nerve was performed according to the Gardner-Robertson hearing classification system [7] (PTA: Pure-Tone-Audiometry) (Table 2) and SDS (Speech-Discrimination Scale) by an oto-laryngologist. PTA was performed on the day of treatment and at the last follow-up. The mean hearing threshold was calculated at the frequencies of 500, 1000, 1500, 2000 and 3000 Hz.

Table 2. *Hearing Function According to Gardner-Robertson [7]*

Grade	Description	Pure-tone-average (decibels)	Speech discrimination score (percent)
I	good to excellent	0–30	70–100
II	servicable	31–50	50–69
III	nonservicable	51–90	5–49
IV	poor	91–100	1–4
V	none	not testable	0

Table 3. *House-Brackmann [10] Scale for Assessment of Facial Nerve Function*

Grade	Description
I	normal in all areas
II	mild dysfunction (slight weakness on close inspection; complete eye closure)
III	moderate dysfunction (obvious but not disfiguring difference between two sides; forehead shows slight to moderate movement; complete eye closure with effort)
IV	moderately severe dysfunction (obvious weakness or disfiguring asymmetry; no forehead movement; incomplete eye closure)
V	severe dysfunction (barely perceptible motion)
VI	total paralysis

Radiosurgical Technique

Assessment for RS was made after MRI-based diagnosis, clinical evaluation and informed consent. All patients were informed about the three treatment possibilities of observation, microsurgery and RS.

Patients were admitted on the day prior to RS. For the procedure an image-compatible Leksell stereotactic coordinate head frame was fixed under local anesthesia. CT/MR-images were obtained using thin slices. Before March 1993 RS was guided by CT scans with 3 mm slices (in the first 17 patients). However, since then, patients underwent RS under the guidance of MR images using 2 mm slices. Several isocenters were identified for use in constructing a radiosurgical plan suitable to the intracanicular and extracanicular components of the tumour. Gamma plan was used to calculate the image-integrated planning of doses. The Gamma Knife Model B was applied for treatment, 201 Cobalt-60-beams being delivered through an interchangeable collimator helmet with beam diameters of 4, 8, 14 or 18 mm. The collimator size selected depended on the location of the lesion and one or more isocenters were used to provide a marginal (30–80%) dose of 10–18 Gy in a single treatment session. Doses delivered to the tumour margin were up to 18 Gy in the early years but were decreased later to an average of 12–14 Gy.

Maximum irradiation exposure of trigeminal and facial nerves did not exceed a maximum of 9 Gy, irradiation to the brain stem was limited to 12 Gy. Patients were discharged from the hospital the day after the procedure.

Results

Within the first 12 hours after RS, 18% of the patients suffered from nausea and/or vomiting, 12%

complained of transient headache. Both symptoms responded well to symptomatic treatment.

Control of tumour growth was achieved in 96%, with a shrinkage occurring in 40% in primary RS. In two cases the schwannoma disappeared completely. In four cases (4%) tumour growth or enlargement of preexisting cystic components was noted. 75% of the treated lesions developed central radionecrosis. In the group that underwent resection previously no further tumour growth was noted. A regression was noted in 25%, a central radionecrosis in 65% of cases.

Neurological evaluations after a follow-up of at least 60 months showed an amelioration of the overall clinical state in 50% of the patients with primary RS compared to 10% who experienced a deterioration of their condition. Loss of hearing and tinnitus remained unchanged in 50% (30 patients). Useful hearing (according to Gardner-Robertson I and II), preradiosurgically documented in this series, could be preserved in 55% of cases (16 patients). In the remaining 45%, gradual loss of useful hearing occurred within 24 months after treatment. A delayed loss of hearing after 36 months was observed in one patient only.

After previous resection, no additional facial nor trigeminal affection was noted. There was no change in audiological parameters in this group. Four patients reported an improvement in tinnitus while another one complained of a worsening condition.

No patient had vagal or glossopharyngeal dysfunction. There were no fatal complications.

No patient described any new neurological problem between 37 and 120 months after the procedure. Detailed informations concerning the preservation of hearing and the facial nerve function are presented in Tables 4–7.

Delayed transient neurological signs comprised mild trigeminal neuropathy (paraesthesia) in five patients (5%) and incomplete facial nerve palsy (according to House-Brackmann II and III) in six patients (6%).

The incomplete facial palsy recovered completely in four but remained in two patients (Table 5). In two female patients who presented with a cystic vestibular schwannoma, a rapid tumour progression was observed at 4 and another at 8 months after RS and subacute microsurgical decompression/evacuation of the cyst was performed. In two cases, hydrocephalus formation necessitated a shunting procedure. Two patients underwent microsurgical decompression due to tumour growth 18 and 24 months after RS, respectively. Six patients developed a transient enlargement

Table 4. *Useful Hearing (Gardner-Robertson I and II) [7] on the Side of the Radiosurgically Treated Lesion after Primary RS*

Number of patients	29	29	20	17	16	16
Months after RS	0	6	12	24	36	60

Table 5. *Function of the Facial Nerve in 60 Patients Before and 60 Months after Primary RS According to House-Brackmann Grade I–VI [10]*

Grade	Before RS	After RS
I	48	46
II	4	5
III	5	6
IV	2	2
V	1	1
VI	0	0
Total	60	60

Table 6. *Characteristics of 40 Patients Before RS (after Previous Microsurgical Decompression): Unchanged CND 60 Months after RS*

Grade	Number of patients	Percent of tumours
Facial nerve function according to House-Brackmann Grade I–VI [10]		
I	10	25
II	8	20
III	4	10
IV	6	15
V	4	10
VI	8	20
Total	40	100
Hearing function according to Gardner-Robertson [7]		
I	0	0
II	3	8
III	6	15
IV	6	15
V	25	62
Total	40	100

Table 7. *Hearing Function According to Gardner-Robertson [7] in Patients with Vestibular Schwannomas Treated by Primnary RS*

Grade	Number of patients	
I	10	5
II	19	11
III	16	23
IV	3	3
V	12	18
Total	60	60

Left: pre-RS, right: 60 months post-RS.

of the ventricular system between 5 and 9 months after RS which was treated symptomatically by steroids.

The group of 17 patients who received treatment based on planning with 3-mm CT slices included two who needed microsurgical decompression, one trigeminal neuropathy, and three of the facial cases. Two transient ventricular enlargements were observed in the group.

Useful (G-R II) or residual hearing (G-R III), preradiosurgically documented in 8% and 15% of the patients with failed microsurgery, respectively, could be preserved (Table 6).

Discussion

In the majority of cases, the "acoustic neuroma" is a vestibular schwannoma originating from the vestibular nerve but only compressing the cochlear nerve. The natural history of vestibular schwannomas is not yet fully understood. Up to 70% of patients exhibit a spontaneous arrest of tumour growth or slower growth over years or even decades [14]. The discussion concerning this matter will not be settled before long-term MR studies are available in a large patient group [2, 16].

In recent years, an increasing number of publications have introduced RS as an effective alternative treatment resulting in both tumour control and good functional outcome [11, 19, 20, 21, 29, 30]. Results following radiosurgical treatment can be considered particularly favourable when compared to patients undergoing a second surgical intervention [20]. On the treatment of recurrent tumours there exist only few articles. Revision surgery is afflicted with major complications like cerebrospinal fluid leak, ataxia, facial nerve palsy, and/or other multiple cranial nerve deficits (CND) [1, 4, 17, 22]. Other authors state that patients with recurrence or evidence of growing tumour following surgery were referred for stereotactic radiosurgery but give no information on the further outcome.

Most investigators reported a high rate of tumour control (growth arrest) or even shrinkage following RS [21, 30, 31]. In accordance with Yamasoba *et al.* [34] we confirmed that preservation or loss of hearing was correlated neither with the initial tumour volume nor with the decrease of tumour size.

Persistent hydrocephalus formation as observed in two patients only is rare and may be due to an elevation of CSF protein level [15, 27]. Samii and Matthies [23] admitted a rise of hydrocephalus in 2.3% of the patients after surgical resection.

Prasad and Steiner [21] state that transient increase in tumour volume may happen within the first year after RS but it should not be assumed to be tumour growth. Instead, it represents swelling as an early change in response to irradiation and should be treated symptomatically by steroids.

Vestibular schwannomas are usually nonspherical shaped tumours. They are preferrably treated by using two or more isocenters and smaller diameter collimators. Flickinger's integrated logistic formula predicted a dramatic lowering of the risks of complication when the target volume is treated with two isocentres instead of one. The radiation dose may be shaped by blocking individual beams [5, 6].

Figure 1 shows a commonly used isodose distribution with two 14 mm collimator isocenters covering the intracerebral portion of the tumour and one 8 mm collimator covering the intracanicular portion. Vestibular schwannomas are regarded as "late-responding targets surrounded by late-responding normal tissue" [12]. Larson states that the dose rises in the interior of the target periphery from perhaps 12 Gy to 24 Gy, whereas beyond the periphery, the dose of the normal tissue drops to insignificant levels. He explains that in a single session the vestibular schwannoma experiences the radiobiologic effect of 100 Gy or more of fractionated radiotherapy, whereas the normal tissue within a narrow rim of a few millimeters from the target experiences the effect of only 10 to 20 Gy of fractionated radiotherapy. He therefore concludes that it is not surprising that benign tumours can be expected to provide excellent progression-free follow-up and clinical responses.

The chance of causing symptomatic radiation injury to the brain by RS is affected dramatically by location. It has long been known that several cranial nerves, especially the optic chiasm/nerves, are more suspectible to injury by fractionated radiation than the rest of the brain. Appearantly there are differences in the effects of radiation in the different cranial nerves. Special sensory nerves (optic and auditory) are the most sensitive, followed by somatic sensory nerves, and then the motor nerves as the least sensitive [5, 13].

In Swedish studies patients were treated and then followed for more than 10 years [15]. Neuropathy of the 5th and 7th cranial nerve, a problem during the first years of RS, could be significantly reduced by a reduction of the dose applied. Doses of 14 Gy to small neurinomas, 12 Gy to medium and 10 Gy to larger respectively, are advocated. By this strategy, perma-

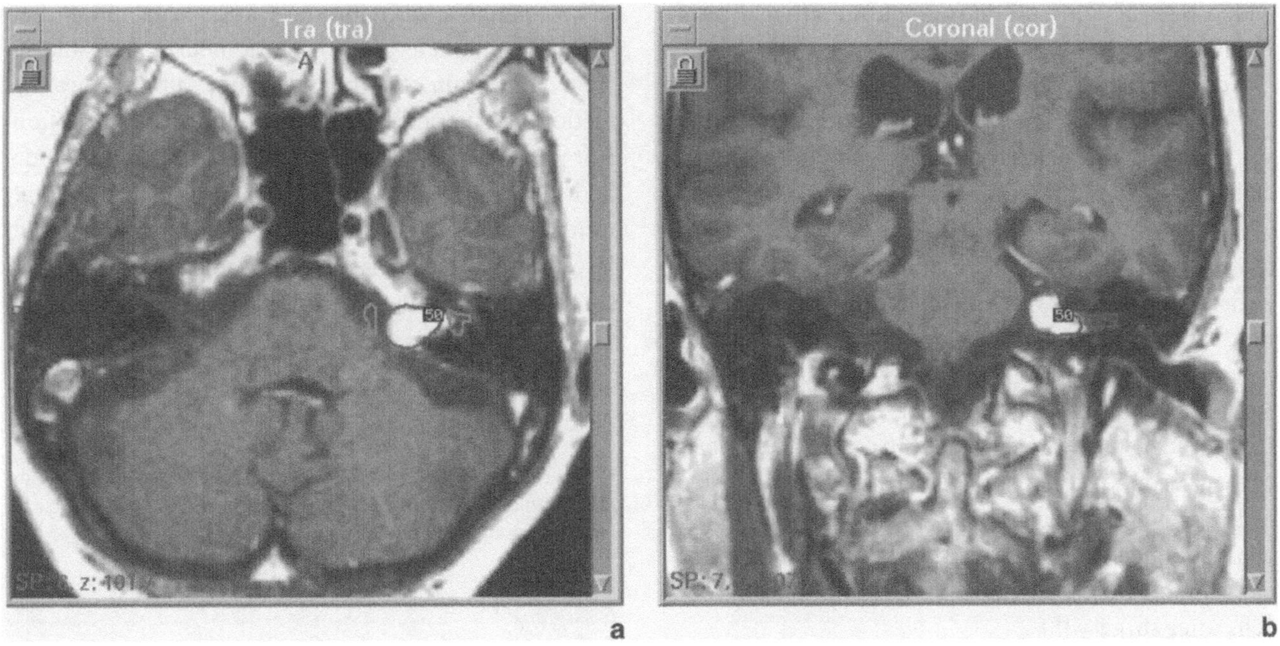

Fig. 1. (a) Axial and (b) Coronal T1-weighted Gadolinium-enhanced MR-images of a 70-year old female patient with left vestibular schwannoma display the 50% isodose (12 Gy) with marked cranial nerves

nent growth control has been obtained in 90% of cases with transient 5th or 7th cranial nerve neuropathy limited to 1–2% of the cases. We confirmed by our own results that with the lowered marginal dose of 12–14 Gy, no differences in tumour control have been observed.

A major part of the complications (such as the 5th and 7th cranial nerve neuropathy) is probably related to a radiation-induced oedema that may be associated with a transient increase in size [21, 30, 31]. Most symptoms were transient, whereas deterioation of hearing, a permanent deficit, was most prominent during the first postradiosurgical year. No significant hearing improvement was observed. None of our patients was left with worse than grade IV facial function.

Several studies compared the outcome in patients with vestibular schwannoma following either microsurgery (MS) or RS [11, 18].

Kondziolka *et al.* [11] emphasized the advantage of the Gamma Knife therapy compared with the outcome of open surgery and observation respectively. They analysed not only the clinical and tumour response but also initiated a survey among radiosurgically treated patients with vestibular schwannoma. Kondziolka compared it to a similiar study by the American Vestibular Schwannoma Association in patients who underwent open surgery [32, 33]. Radiosurgically treated patients favored this treatment modality, especially those who had undergone surgery previously because of a lower rate of complications. 76% of the patients had quickly returned to normal daily life activities. Less neuropsychological problems such as dizziness, sleep disturbance, fatigue and depression were considered favourable features associated with RS. 95% of patients stated that they would recommend the procedure to a friend.

RS conceivably may induce malignant transformation of the tumour or cause new tumours although this is an unproven allegation [3, 9, 25, 26, 28].

Some reports stated that costs of RS are considerably less than those associated with MS, both in terms of direct costs and the indirect costs of lost work days, etc. Following RS, most patients are able to return to work within 7 days [18, 19, 21].

Although excellent results after microsurgery are published by various authors, still there exists no ideal surgical approach (suboccipital/translabyrinthine/middle fossa). Recent surgical series report that within several years of surgery 2–5% of patients have a recurrence. While Samii and Matthies [23, 24] performed complete tumour removal in 98% of cases with recurrence only in 0.7% (6 of 880 patients), information from the Acoustic Neuroma Registry [32, 33] shows that 8% of patients with follow-up MRI have either residual or recurrent tumour one year after surgery. A wide range of tumour recurrence after surgical resection was therefore reported.

Cerullo *et al.* [1] stated that, using survival analysis, 19% of the patients experienced a recurrence within 7.5 years of surgery. Therefore, recurrence following so-called complete tumour removal is a clinical problem.

In their study on regrowth of residual neurinoma after surgery Ohta *et al.* [17] pointed out that in most patients anatomical preservation of the nerve could not be obtained without leaving tumour overlying the nerve. The facial nerve is flattened by compression of the tumour, and its sheath is densely adherent to the tumour capsule around the porus. For this reason tumour around this area may be deliberately left so as to keep anatomical continuity of the facial nerve. Histopathological observations suggest that all anatomically intact facial nerves may harbour schwannoma cells after surgery [8].

An important fact seems to be complete tumour removal from the fundus to the porus of the internal acoustic meatus. This procedure might disrupt the blood suppy to the growing origin of the tumour, which would lead to no tumour regrowth after the operation [4, 8, 17].

Cerullo *et al.* [1] found some other interesting aspects on vestibular schwannoma recurrence that patients with tumours equal to or larger than 3 cm had a significantly decreased risk of recurrence than those with smaller tumours. Pollock and coworkers report in their series that radiosurgery proved to be a safe and effective alternative to additional microsurgery in patients in whom the initial microsurgical removal failed. The high percentage of CND before radiosurgery in our series might be explained by surgical complications or the recurrence itself and is similar to findings in other series [20].

We advocate RS as a safe and effective treatment modality as Pollock and coworkers did. No new cranial nerve neuropathy was noted in our group.

Conclusion

Vestibular schwannomas may be treated by different options: MS, RS and observation. Benefits associated with RS include short hospital stay, reduction in hospital-based charges and rapid return to preoperative functional status or employment. Useful hearing and good cranial nerve function may be preserved and is comparable to MS.

For patients with tumours measuring more than 30 mm in diameter and/or cystic neurinomas and lesions with brain stem compression, microsurgical resection at experienced centers is the preferred option. For patients harboring small to medium sized tumours and intracanicular tumours, RS is a therapeutical alternative. RS should be considered for all patients who have a progression of previously microsurgically subtotal resected vestibular schwannomas.

Acknowledgments

We appreciate the contributions of our physicists Helmut Guss and Karlheinz Feichtinger and the sophisticated work of Ms. Elfriede Meier in preparing the manuscript.

References

1. Cerullo L, Grutsch J, Osterdock R (1998) Recurrence of vestibular (acoustic) schwannomas in surgical patients where preservation of facial and cochlear nerve is the priority. Br J Neurosurg 12: 547–552
2. Charabi S, Thomsen J, Mantoni M, Charabi B, Jorgensen B, Borgesen SE, Gyldensted C, Tos M (1995) Acoustic neuroma (vestibular schwannoma): growth and surgical and nonsurgical consequences of the wait-and-see policy. Otolaryngol Head Neck Surg 113: 5–14
3. Comey CH, Mc Laughlin MR, Jho HD, Martinez AJ, Lunsford LD (1998) Death from a malignant cerebellopontine angle triton tumour despite stereotactic radiosurgery. J Neurosurg 89: 653–658
4. El-Kashlan HK, Zeitoun H, Arts HA, Hoff JT, Telian SA (2000) Recurrence of acoustic neuroma after incomplete resection. Am J Otol 21: 389–392
5. Flickinger JC, Kondziolka D, Lunsford LD (1996) Dose and diameter relationships for facial, trigeminal, and acoustic neuropathies following acoustic neuroma radiosurgery. Radiother Oncol 41: 215–219
6. Flickinger JC, Kondziolka D, Lunsford LD (1999) Dose selection in stereotactic radiosurgery. Neurosurg Clin North Am 10: 271–280
7. Gardner G, Robertson JH (1988) Hearing preservation in unilateral acoustic neuroma surgery. Ann Otol Rhinol Laryngol 97: 55–66
8. Haberkamp TJ, Meyer GA, Fox M (1998) Surgical exposure of the fundus of the internal auditory canal: anatomic limits of the middle fossa versus the retrosigmoid transcanal approach. Laryngoscope 108: 1190–1194
9. Hanabusa K, Morikawa A, Murata T, Taki W (2001) Acoustic neuroma with malignant transformation. Case report. J Neurosurg 95: 518–521
10. House JW, Brackmann DE (1985) Facial nerve grading system. Otolaryngol Head Neck Surg 93: 146–147
11. Kondziolka D, Lunsford LD, MC Laughlin MR, Flickinger JC (1998) Long-term outcomes after radiosurgery for acoustic neuromas. N Engl J Med 339: 1426–1433
12. Larson DA, Flickinger JC, Loeffler JS (1993) The radiobiology of radiosurgery. Int J Radiat Oncol Biol Phys 25: 557–561

13. Linskey ME, Flickinger JC, Lunsford LD (1993) Cranial nerve length predicts the risk of delayed facial and trigeminal neuropathies after acoustic tumour stereotactic radiosurgery. Int J Radiat Oncol Biol Phys 25: 227–233
14. Niemczyk K, Vaneecloo FM, Lemaitre L, Lejeune JP, Skarzynski H, Dubrulle F, Vincent C (1999) The growth of acoustic neuromas in volumetric radiologic assessment. Am J Otol 20: 244–248
15. Noren G (1998) Long-term complications following gamma knife radiosurgery of vestibular schwannomas. Stereotact Funct Neurosurg 70 [Suppl] 1: 65–73
16. O'Donoghue GM, Nikopoulos T, Thomsen J (1999) Management of acoustic neuroma. N Engl J Med 340: 1120–1121
17. Ohta S, Yokoyama T, Nishizawa S, Uemura K (1998) Regrowth of the residual tumour after acoustic neurinoma surgery. Br J Neurosurg 12: 419–422
18. Ott K (1996) A comparison of craniotomy and gamma knife charges in a community-based gamma knife center. Stereotact Funct Neurosurg 66 [Suppl] 1: 357–364
19. Pollock BE, Lunsford LD, Noren G (1998) Vestibular schwannoma management in the next century: a radiosurgical perspective. Neurosurgery 43: 475–483
20. Pollock BE, Lunsford LD, Flickinger JC, Clyde BL, Kondziolka D (1998) Vestibular schwannoma management. Part I. Failed microsurgery and the role of delayed stereotactic radiosurgery. J Neurosurg 89: 944–948
21. Prasad D, Steiner M, Steiner L (2000) Gamma surgery for vestibular schwannoma. J Neurosurg 92: 745–759
22. Robertson JB Jr, Brackmann DE, Hitselberger WE (1996) Acoustic neuroma recurrence after suboccipital resection: management with translabyrinthine resection. Am J Otol 17: 307–311
23. Samii M, Matthies C (1997) Management of 1000 vestibular schwannomas (acoustic neuromas): surgical management and results with an emphasis on complications and how to avoid them. Neurosurgery 40: 11–21
24. Samii M, Matthies C (1997) Management of 1000 vestibular schwannomas (acoustic neuromas): hearing function in 1000 tumour resections. Neurosurgery 40: 248–262
25. Slattery WH III, Brackmann DE (1995) Results of surgery following stereotactic irradiation for acoustic neuromas. Am J Otol 16: 315–321
26. Thompson BG, Coffey RJ, Flickinger JC, Lunsford LD (1990) Stereotactic radiosurgery of small intracranial tumours: neuropathological correlation in three patients. Surg Neurol 33: 96–104
27. Thomsen J, Tos M, Borgesen SE (1990) Gamma knife: hydrocephalus as a complication of stereotactic radiosurgical treatment of an acoustic neuroma. Am J Otol 11: 330–333
28. Thomsen J, Mirz F, Wetke R, Astrup J, Bojsen-Moller M, Nielsen E (2000) Intracranial sarcoma in a patient with neurofibromatosis type 2 treated with gamma knife radiosurgery for vestibular schwannoma. Am J Otol 21: 364–370
29. Unger F, Walch C, Papaefthymiou G, Trummer M, Eustacchio S, Pendl G (1999) Die Radiochirurgie des Akustikusneurinoms als minimal-invasive Alternative zur Mikrochirurgie. HNO 47: 1046–1051
30. Unger F, Walch C, Papaefthymiou G, Eustacchio S, Feichtinger K, Quehenberger F, Pendl G (2002) Long-term results of radiosurgery for vestibular schwannomas. Zentralbl Neurochir (in press)
31. Valentino V, Raimondi AJ (1995) Tumour response and morphological changes of acoustic neurinomas after radiosurgery. Acta Neurochir (Wien) 133: 157–163
32. Wiegand DA, Fickel V (1989) Acoustic neuroma – the patient's perspective: subjective assessment of symptoms, diagnosis, therapy, and outcome in 541 patients. Laryngoscope 99: 179–187
33. Wiegand DA, Ojemann RG, Fickel V (1996) Surgical treatment of acoustic neuroma (vestibular schwannoma) in the United States: report from the acoustic neuroma registry. Laryngoscope 106: 58–66
34. Yamasoba T, Kurita H, Ito K, Mizuno M, Nakamura M, Sugasawa M, Sugasawa K, Sasaki T (1996) Auditory findings after stereotactic radiosurgery in acoustic neurinoma. Skull Base Surg 6: 163–167

Correspondence: M. O. Frank Unger, Department of Neurosurgery, Karl-Franzens University, Auenbruggerplatz 29, A-8036 Graz, Austria.

Acta Neurochir (2002) [Suppl] 84: 85–90

Gamma Knife Radiosurgery of Brainstem Gliomas

I. Fuchs, W. Kreil, B. Sutter, G. Papaethymiou, and **G. Pendl**

Department of Neurosurgery, Karl-Franzens University, Graz, Austria

Summary

From August 1992 until December 1999 Gamma Knife radiosurgery (GKRS) was applied to 21 patients (male to female ratio 14:7) with brainstem gliomas. Patient's median age was 23 years (8–56 years). All tumours were histologically confirmed by biopsy or open surgery: 12 low-grade gliomas and 9 malignant growths. Two lesions were located primarily in the medulla, 12 in the pons and 7 in the midbrain. A median dose of 12 Gy (9–20 Gy) was applied to the tumour margin by the median isodose of 45%. Prior to radiosurgery 4 patients were treated by conventional radiotherapy, 1 had radiotherapy and chemotherapy, 1 patient underwent chemotherapy, and 1 patient was shunted due to hydrocephalus.

Neuroimaging controls (MR, CT) were obtained from 19 patients. The median interval between radiosurgery and the last neuroimaging control was 11.8 months (1–74 months). Neuroimaging depicted tumour progression in 2 patients, stable disease in 10 patients and regression in 3 cases. Follow-up periods ranged between 3 and 99 months (median 29 months). The neurological state improved in 5 patients. Microsurgical cyst fenestration was performed in 1 patient after GKRS, shunting procedure was necessary for 2 patients. Nine patients died unrelated to radiosurgery within 3 to 45 months (median 20.7 months).

GKRS is an effective treatment modality for brainstem gliomas with satisfying tumour control and functional outcome.

Keywords: Brainstem; Gamma Knife; glioma; radiosurgery.

Introduction

Brainstem gliomas are uncommon tumours with an incidence of about 2% of all brain tumours, but approximately 10 to 25% of brain tumours in children [5, 6, 21, 22, 25]. High morbidity and mortality rates associated with tumour growth in this location forces considerations to treat patients presenting with a brainstem glioma. Despite advances and refinements in microsurgical techniques some eloquent areas of the brain still remain unaccessible for surgery due to unacceptable morbidity and mortality [4]. Lesions located in the brainstem are still regarded as major challenge to neurosurgery. Radical removal cannot be achieved in most cases [12]. Radiosurgery has become a well accepted adjuvant treatment alternative to reduce the risk and to improve the outcome at the same time.

Patients and Methods

Between August 1992 and December 1999, 21 patients with gliomas located in the brainstem were treated by stereotactic radiosurgery using the 201-source Cobalt-60 Gamma Knife Model B at the Department of Neurosurgery, Karl-Franzens University, Graz. The brain stem was defined as including the midbrain, pons and medulla oblongata. The age of these patients ranged from 8 to 56 years (median 23 years). The male to female ratio was 2:1. The distribution of the tumour location is listed in table 1 and demonstrates a predominance in the pons [24]. Nineteen patients presented with brainstem signs, 2 patients suffered only from cephalgia. The most common sign was hemiparesis, followed by ataxia, diplopia and cranial nerve deficit (Table 2). One patient underwent shunting procedure prior to radiosurgery.

For the procedure an image-compatible Leksell stereotactic coordinate head frame was fixed under local anaesthesia in all but one patient (an 8-year-old child who had general anaesthesia). CT/MR-images were obtained using thin slices. Till March 1993 radiosurgery was guided by contrast enhanced CT scans with 3 mm slices (in the first 2 patients) and since then patients underwent radiosurgery under the guidance of gadolinium-enhanced MR-images with 2 mm slices. The appropriate isodose configuration, total dosage, number of isocenters and treatment time were calculated according to the planning software (Gamma Plan®). Various collimator sizes – 4, 8, 14 or 18 mm – had been selected depending on the location, configuration and volume of the lesion. Before and after GKRS caliber measurements in three separate dimensions were performed. Volumetry was calculated at the time of GKRS.

Table 1. *Location of 21 Brainstem Gliomas Treated by GKRS*

	Benign gliomas n = 12	Malignant gliomas n = 9
Midbrain	5	2
Pons	6	6
Medulla oblongata	1	1

Benign Gliomas

Twelve patients (9 male and 3 female) with low-grade gliomas underwent stereotactic GKRS. In 4 cases (33.3%) they corresponded to grade I and in 8 cases (66.6%) to grade II of the World Health Organisation (WHO) tumour classification system [14]. Age ranged from 8 to 56 years (median 23 years). Ten patients had microsurgery for tumour resection 1 to 3 times prior to radiosurgery, 2 patients had stereotactic biopsy. One patient had been previously subject to a shunting procedure. The mean period between surgery and GKRS was 2 months (0.4–41.5 months). Two patients had fractioned radiotherapy with a total dose of 60 Gy, and 1 patient underwent chemotherapy prior to GKRS. The minimal dose to the tumour margin was dependent on location, volume of the lesion and prior radiation therapy. Tumour volumes of 0.27–15.39 ccm were covered by marginal doses ranging from 9 to 20 Gy (mean 12 Gy) using 1–10 isocenters (median 3). According to large tumour size, one patient underwent a staged radiosurgical treatment with an interval of 1.6 months.

Malignant Gliomas

The mean age in 9 patients (5 male, 4 female) with malignant gliomas was 43 years (14–54 years). Histological specimens were obtained by 10 surgical procedures (7 tumour resections and 3 biopsies) and revealed grade III gliomas for 6 patients and grade IV gliomas for the remaining 3 patients. Adjacent fenestration of a tumour cyst was also performed in 1 patient after microsurgical tumour resection. Fractioned radiotherapy with 60 Gy was performed in 2 patients, and 1 patient received radiotherapy with 54 Gy combined with chemotherapy, prior to GKRS. Time interval between last surgery and GKRS was 0.3–37.9 months (median 1.2 months). The median tumour volume was 5.1 ccm (0.88–39 ccm). The median marginal dose delivered by 2–7 isocenters (median 5) to an average isodose volume of 45% (40–65%) was 15 Gy (10–20 Gy).

Table 2. *Neurological Symptoms in 21 Patients with Brainstem Gliomas before GKRS*

Symptoms	No. of patients
Hemiparesis	7
Ataxia	6
Cranial nerve deficit	6*
– 4th cranial nerve	1
– 5th cranial nerve	1
– 6th cranial nerve	2
– 7th cranial nerve	3
– 10th cranial nerve	1
Diplopia	6
Dysarthria	2
Cephalgia	2
Dysphagia	1
Strabism	1
Aphasia	1
Epilepsy	1

* More than one nerve was affected in 2 patients.

Results

Follow-up comprises neurological status, including Karnofsky performance rating, as well as neuroimaging by MRT or contrast-enhanced CT [21] (Table 3).

Benign Gliomas

Postradiosurgically 36 follow-up scans revealed tumour growth control in 11 patients with shrinkage in 6 cases, and only in 1 case tumour enlargement could be observed. A mean follow-up period of 41 months (3.5–99 months) disclosed a stable neurological status in 3 cases, ameliorated status in 4 cases (Fig. 1), and worsening in 2 cases. Three patients died after 3.5–27.6 months (median 20.7 months) due to their general condition, unrelated to radiosurgery. Shunting procedure became necessary for two patients after radiosurgery.

Malignant Gliomas

From 8 of 9 patients 24 neuroimaging scans were available after radiosurgery. These follow-up scans presented smaller tumours in 2 cases, stable sizes in 5 cases and enlargement in 1 case. Three patients suffering from multiloculated glioblastoma died within 3 to 5.8 months (median 5.5 months), 3 patients with anaplastic astrocytoma died after a median interval of 28 months (23.7–45 months). Tumour growth outside the radiosurgical treatment volume as well as poor clinical condition were seen in these 6 cases. The clinical con-

Table 3. *Results in 21 Patients with Brainstem Gliomas Treated by GKRS*

Tumour size after GKRS					Clinical status after GKRS			
	No neuroimaging	Absent or smaller	No change	Larger	Improved	Stable	Worse	Dead
Benign gliomas n = 12	–	6	5	1	4	3	2	3
Malignant gliomas n = 9	1	2	5	1	1	2	–	6

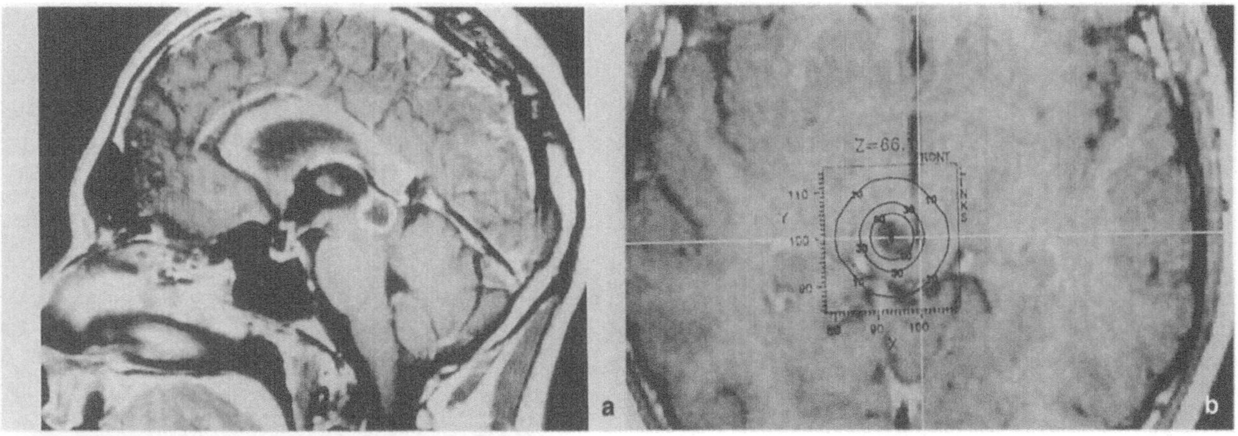

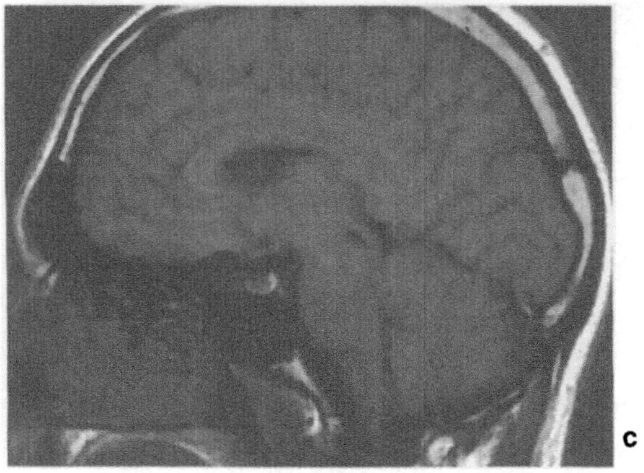

Fig. 1. (a) T1-weighted gadolinium-enhanced cranial MRI showing a grade II astrocytoma before surgery in a 24-year-old patient with ataxia. (b) The borderline of the resection cavity was enclosed within the 60% isodose line. As a marginal dose 14 Gy were delivered to a treatment volume of 0.27 ccm. The clinical condition improved slightly after treatment. (c) Follow-up scans after 6 years showing no evidence of recurrence

dition of the remaining 3 patients improved in 1 case and was stable in 2 cases after a median follow-up period of 74 months (24–98 months). One of these patients, who had undergone implantation of a drainage into a tumour cyst prior to craniotomy and radiosurgery, developed malfunction of the drainage and regrowth of the tumour cyst: In this male patient microsurgical cyst fenestration 18 months after radiosurgery had been performed. Seventy four months after radiosurgery he still is in a satisfying clinical condition. (Fig. 2). No therapy related mortality occurred and no patient suffered serious morbidity after GKRS. Within the first 12 hours after radiosurgery, one third of the patients suffered from nausea, vomiting and/or transient headache. These symptoms responded well to symptomatic treatment.

Discussion

Modern microsurgery, including intraoperative brainstem evoked responses and neuronavigation improved surgical results, nevertheless surgical treatment of tumours within the brainstem is still associated with a marked degree of morbidity and mortality [19, 20]. The localisation and histological nature of the brainstem lesions are important factors concerning postoperative morbidity and mortality [1, 6, 8, 9, 19, 23, 24, 25, 26]. For low-grade gliomas complete resection is the ideal treatment, if that is not possible, at least reduction of tumour mass should be aimed [2, 19, 20, 21].

In recent years, an increasing number of publications have introduced radiosurgery as an effective method for tumour control with good functional outcome in brainstem tumours [3, 7, 10, 11, 13, 15, 16, 17]. Tumour control of brainstem lesions is an important issue for extending survival time and improving quality of life.

Huang *et al.* presented radiosurgery for brainstem metastases. For these well demarcated lesions they applied a median marginal dose of 16 Gy (12–20 Gy). Local tumour control rate in 95% of patients could be achieved. Although the minimum effective radiosurgical dose to the tumour is not known, a minimum dose of 11 Gy to the margin of a brainstem tumour should be used according to the opinion of the authors. Nevertheless marginal dose of 20 Gy to the brainstem parenchyma had been save in their experience [11].

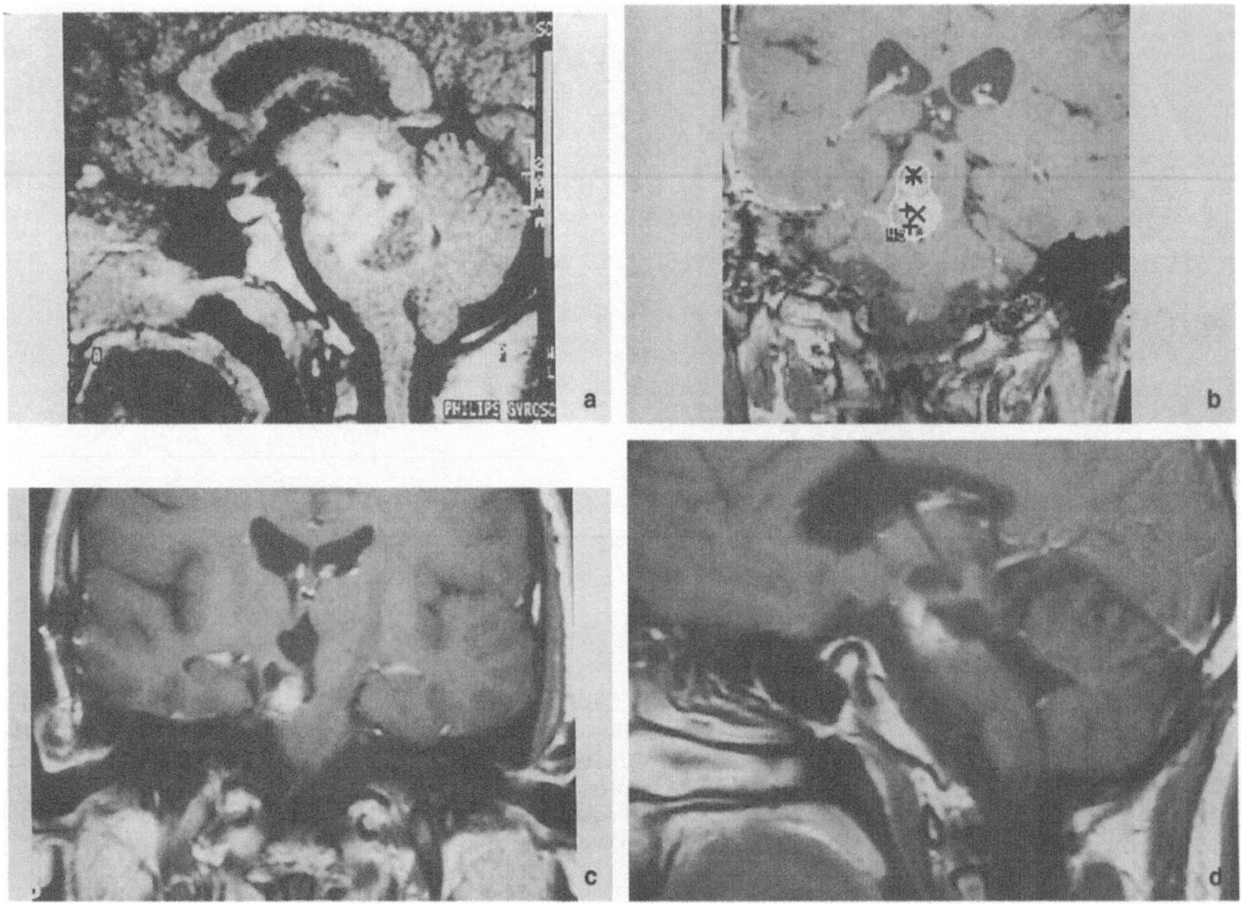

Fig. 2. (a) T1-weighted gadolinium-enhanced cranial MR-image (sagittal view) displaying a right-sided brainstem astrocytoma grade III in a 16-year-old patient with a history of right-sided hemiparesis and seizures. Biopsy and radiation followed by cyst drainage and microsurgical reoperation were performed prior to radiosurgery. (b) Four years after the first therapy a treatment volume of 8.5 ccm was covered by a marginal dose of 10 Gy at the 45% isodose line. During postradiosurgical course the tumour cyst was drained operatively again. (c/d) Latest MR-image, obtained 74 months after GKRS, demonstrating reduced tumour size. Clinically, the hemiparesis improved and the patient is doing well

Hirato *et al.* reported 10 patients with brainstem tumours of different dignity with marginal doses ranging from 12.1 to 13.5 Gy. In 2 cases of radiosurgically treated gliomas, they indicated little or no response to treatment. They saw patient's death after 7 months in one case and a second patient alive after 1 year follow-up. One patient with cystic growth of a glioma after GKRS was treated by surgery [19].

For brainstem AVMs, Massager *et al.* used marginal doses ranging from 11.5 to 30 Gy without negative side effects on the surrounding area [18].

A dose as high as 20 Gy to the tumour margin has been save in our own experience nevertheless in current practice we limit the marginal dose to 16 Gy.

Some authors report a good local tumour control of low-grade gliomas after stereotactic radiosurgery [3, 7, 10, 13, 16, 17].

Kida *et al.* achieved tumour control in 91.7% of their radiosurgically treated grade I astrocytomas as well as volume reduction in 50%, for grade II astrocytomas. They also attained volume reduction in 46.2% and tumour control in 87.2% after a mean follow-up period of 27.6 months. Radiation-induced oedema in 35.2%, cyst formation or cyst enlargement in 9.8% and transient tumour enlargement in 5.9% of their patients are described. The mean marginal dose for the treatment of grade I gliomas they applied was 12.5 Gy and for grade II gliomas 15.7 Gy [13].

Baracia *et al.* report about their radiosurgical treatment of 16 patients with deeply seated low-grade gliomas with a conventional gamma source. Although they attained good clinical results for 13 of their patients with disappearance of the tumour in 50%, diminishing in size in 13% and stop of growing in 31%, 3 patients with brainstem tumours and poor condition before treatment deteriorated [3].

In our own series no radiation induced oedema occurred, cystic growth was seen in one patient and one other had tumour growth and died 3.5 months after radiosurgery.

Grabb *et al.* see radiosurgery alone as save and effective treatment modality for unresectable benign glial tumours of childhood as well as an adjuvant treatment for unresectable malignant gliomas. Marginal doses ranging from 11 to 20 Gy were administered at the 50 to 60% isodose lines. Eighty-eight percent of unresectable benign neoplasm's were controlled by radiosurgery, whereas 8% of malignant neoplasms were controlled. All tumours were deep seated. Four children developed neurological signs or symptoms attributable to radiosurgery, increased peritumoural edema was seen in 6 children [7]. These results, as well as the authors' own experience are in contradistinction to the work of Hirato *et al.* who require a fractionated treatment as an alternative for the treatment of brainstem gliomas. In their 2 cases they report an unpleasant outcome [10].

Legat *et al.* report of Gamma-Knife radiosurgery of 11 patients with benign and 12 patients with malignant midline gliomas. Peripheral doses with a range of 10–22 Gy to benign and 9–30 Gy to malignant gliomas had been administered. For the benign tumours a local control in 78% of the patients had been achieved. Patients with glioblastomas had a mean survival time of 6 months. Tumour control for grade III astrocytomas was achieved in 75%. No serious morbidity related to GKRS was described [16].

Kondziolka *et al.* treated patients with high grade gliomas. Tumours with mean diameters smaller than 3.5 cm at any brain location could be covered by isodose volumes. For glioblastomas they applied a median marginal dose of 15.5 Gy mostly by the 50% isodose line. Anaplastic astrocytomas received a mean dose of 15.2 Gy also by the 50% isodose line in 90% of cases. In their series with 64 patients suffering from glioblastoma and 43 patients with anaplastic astrocytoma they saw an improved survival benefit after radiosurgery for both patient groups. Intravenously administered chemotherapy in addition to radiosurgery did not bring any improvement for these patients. The median survival time after radiosurgery for glioblastoma patients was 16 months after treatment, for patients with anaplastic astrocytomas 32 months. They conclude that boost stereotactic surgery is a save and potentially effective treatment for these patients [15].

In our series patients with glioblastomas in the brainstem seem not to profit from radiosurgery concerning survival periods, whereas patients with anaplastic astrocytomas in the brainstem seem to achieve longer survival periods.

In their report of 31 patients who had radiosurgery for glioblastomas Masciopinto *et al.* do not see a benefit for stereotactic radiosurgery over traditional surgery (or biopsy) and regional radiation. For treatment they applied does ranging from 10 to 20 Gy at 40 to 90% peripheral isodose lines with the linear accelerator [17].

Conclusions

Although partial resection of brainstem gliomas by microsurgery may often be a viable option, radical resection of these lesions in most cases cannot be achieved without neurological deficits and morbidity for the patients.

In these cases GKRS seems to be an important adjuvant therapy to modern neurosurgical techniques.

References

1. Albright AL, Guthkelch AN, Packer RJ, Price RA, Rourke LB (1986) Prognostic factors in pediatric brain-stem gliomas. J Neurosurg 65: 751–755
2. Alvisi C, Cerisoli M, Maccheroni ME (1985) Long-term results of surgically treated brainstem gliomas. Acta Neurochir (Wien) 76: 12–17
3. Barcia JA, Barcia-Salorio JL, Ferrer C, Ferrer E, Algas R, Hernandez G (1994) Stereotactic radiosurgery of deeply seated low grade gliomas. Acta Neurochir (Wien) [Suppl] 62: 58–61
4. Chang WH, Kak VK, Banerjee AK, Rajwanshi A (1990) Stereotaxic biopsy of brain-stem tumours in children. Childs Nerv Syst 6: 409–411
5. Cloughesi TF, Black KL (1994) Diagnosis and management of brainstem gliomas. Neurosurg Q 4: 174–186
6. Epstein F, Farmer JP (1993) Brain-stem glioma growth patterns. J Neurosurg 78: 408–412
7. Grabb PA, Lunsford LD, Albright AL, Kondziolka D, Flickinger JC (1996) Stereotactic radiosurgery for glial neoplasms of childhood. Neurosurgery 38: 696–701
8. Grigsby PW, Garcia DM, Simpson JR, Fineberg BB, Schwartz HG (1989) Prognostic factors and results of therapy for adult thalamic and brainstem tumors. Cancer 63: 2124–2129
9. Heffez DS, Zinreich SJ, Long DM (1990) Surgical resection of intrinsic brain stem lesions: an overview. Neurosurgery 27: 789–798
10. Hirato M, Nakamura M, Inoue HK, Ohye C, Hirato J, Shibazaki T, Andou Y (1995) Gamma knife radiosurgery for the treatment of brainstem tumors. Stereotact Funct Neurosurg 64 [Suppl] 1: 32–41
11. Huang CF, Kondziolka D, Flickinger JC, Lunsford LD (1999) Stereotactic radiosurgery of brainstem metastases. J Neurosurg 91: 563–568

12. Kaplan AM, Albright AL, Zimmerman RA, Roke LB, Li H, Boyett JM, Finlay JL, Wara WM, Packer RJ (1996) Brainstem gliomas in children. Pediatr Neurosurg 24: 185–192
13. Kida Y, Kobayashi T, Mori Y (2000) Gamma knife radiosurgery for low-grade astrocytomas: Results of long-term follow up. J Neurosurg [Suppl] 3 93: 42–46
14. Kleihues P, Cavenee WK (1997) Pathology and genetics of tumours of the nervous system. International Agency for Research on Cancer, France, pp 1–36
15. Kondziolka D, Flickinger JC, Bissonette DJ, Bozik M, Lunsford LD (1997) Survival benefit of stereotactic radiosurgery for patients with malignant glial neoplasms. Neurosurgery 41: 776–785
16. Legat J, Mokry M, Leber K, Schröttner O, Pendl G (1998) Gamma Knife radiosurgery for midline lesions. Kitakanto Med J (S1): 41–50
17. Masciopinto JE, Levin AB, Mehta MP, Rhode BS (1995) Stereotactic radiosurgery for glioblastoma: a final report of 31 patients. J Neurosurg 82: 530–535
18. Massager N, Regis J, Kondziolka D, Njee T, Leviver M (2000) Gamma knife radiosurgery for brainstem arteriovenous malformations: preliminary results. J Neurosurg [Suppl] 3 93: 102–103
19. Pendl G, Vorkapic P, Koniyama M (1990) Microsurgery of midbrain lesions. Neurosurgery 26: 641–648
20. Pendl G, Vorkapic P (1991) Microsurgery of intrinsic midbrain lesions. Acta Neurochir (Wien) [Suppl] 53: 137–143
21. Pool LJ (1968) Gliomas in the region of brain stem. J Neurosurg 29: 164–167
22. Selvapandian S, Rajshekar V, Chandy MJ (1999) Brainstem glioma: Comparative study of clinico-radiological presentation, pathology and outcome in children and adults. Acta Neurochir (Wien) 141: 721–727
23. Smith RR, Zimmerman RA, Packer RJ, Hackney DB, Bilaniuk LT, Sutton LN, Goldberg HI, Grossman RI, Schut L (1990) Pediatric brainstem glioma. Post-radiation clinical and MR follow-up. Neuroradiology 32: 265–271
24. Steck J, Friedman WA (1995) Stereotactic biopsy of brainstem mass lesions. Surg Neurol 43: 563–568
25. Pollack IF, Hoffman HJ, Humphreys RP, Becker L (1993) The long-term outcome after surgical treatment of dorsally exophytic brain-stem gliomas. J Neurosurg 78: 859–863
26. Wang C, Zhang J, Liu A, Sun B, Zhao Y (2000) Surgical treatment of primary midbrain gliomas. Surg Neurol 53: 41–51

Correspondence: Ingo Fuchs, M.D., Department of Neurosurgery, Karl-Franzens University, Auenbruggerplatz 29, 8036 Graz, Austria.

Acta Neurochir (2002) [Suppl] 84: 91–97

The Role of Gamma Knife Radiosurgery in the Management of Glomus Jugulare Tumours

S. Eustacchio, M. Trummer, F. Unger, O. Schröttner, B. Sutter, and **G. Pendl**

Department of Neurosurgery, Karl-Franzens University, Graz, Austria

Summary

Background. Glomus jugulare tumours are usually managed by microsurgical resection and/or radiotherapy with considerable risk for treatment-related morbidity. The role of Gamma Knife Radiosurgery (GKRS) in the management of these lesions remains to be defined.

Method. Between May 1992 and November 2000, 19 patients with glomus tumours underwent GKRS at our department. Nine patients received radiosurgery for residual or recurrent paragangliomas following microsurgical resection and in 10 cases GKRS was performed as primary treatment. The median tumour volume was 5.22 ccm (range: 0,38–33.5 ccm). Marginal doses of 12–20 Gy (median 14 Gy) were applied to enveloping isodose volume curves (Range: 30–55%, median 50%).

Findings. Except for an 81-year-old patient who died 9 months after radiosurgery the observation time ranged from 1.5 to 10 years (median 7.2 yrs). The total tumour control rate was 94.7% (7 cases with decreased and 11 with stable tumour size). The only patient with tumour progression (5,3%) underwent repeated radiosurgical treatment 85 months after initial GKRS. A newly diagnosed second lesion in the cavernous sinus was treated radiosurgically as well 53 months after the first Gamma Knife procedure. On clinical examination 10 patients (52,6%) presented with improved and 8 patients (42,1%) with unchanged neurological status. Deterioration in one patient (5,3%) was not related to tumour or radiosurgery.

Interpretation. As GKRS demonstrated to be a minimally invasive treatment alternative to microsurgery and radiotherapy with no acute or chronic toxicity it should be considered more frequently in the primary or adjuvant strategy for glomus jugulare tumours.

Keywords: Gamma knife; stereotactic radiosurgery; glomus jugulare tumour; paragangliomas.

Introduction

The current treatment options for glomus jugulare tumours are multifold comprising surgical resection, radiotherapy and endovascular occlusion of feeding vessels either in combination or alone [3, 9, 12, 14, 23, 26, 28]. However, the choice of primary therapy remains highly controversial [3, 4, 12–14, 18, 26, 28]. Excision of even small lesions can produce clinically significant sequelae, including Cranial Nerve Deficit (CND), stroke and death [1, 2, 10–12, 18–20, 25, 27, 28]. Embolisation alone does not prevent further tumour progression [20, 21]. Primary radiation therapy cannot guarantee local control of disease and is associated with considerable risk for treatment-related morbidity [3, 4, 14, 22, 26].

The use of Gamma Knife Radiosurgery (GKRS) in the management of patients with glomus jugulare tumours has been sporadically discussed in the literature [5, 6, 9, 13, 15–17, 23]. In this study we assess the outcomes of 19 patients who received GKRS for their newly diagnosed, residual or recurrent jugulare foramen paragangliomas. This represents the largest series reported to date.

Methods and Material

Between May 1992 and November 2000, 19 patients (13 females and 6 males) with glomus jugulare tumours underwent stereotactic radiosurgical treatment using the Leksell Model B Gamma Knife at the Department of Neurosurgery, Karl-Franzens University of Graz, Austria. The age of these patients ranged from 21 to 80 years (median 56 years). Tumour staging according to the system of Glasscock/Jackson 28 is shown in Table 1, while Table 2 displays the distribution of tumour extent using the classification of Fisch 18. In 9 patients GKRS was performed 2.1–120.9 months after microsurgical resection (median 44.5 months) to prevent progression of recurrent or residual glomus tumours. Histologically, they were classified as benign paraganglioma in 7 cases and malignant paraganglioma in two cases. One patient with an incompletely removed tumour had received conventional radiotherapy three years before Gamma Knife treatment. Ten patients were treated by GKRS alone, as they were elderly, medically infirm or declined microsurgical resection. In these cases diagnosis was based on characteristic findings on computed tomography (CT), magnetic resonance imaging (MRI) and four-vessel angiography. Six patients underwent endovascular tumour embolisation 0.1 to 1 month (median 0.1 month) prior to

Table 1. *Distribution of Tumour Type in 19 Patients with Glomus Jugulare Tumours According to the Staging System of Glasscock and Jackson [28]*

Glasscock & Jackson grade	Primary GKRS	Secondary GKRS	Total
I	–	–	–
II	4	3	7
III	4	2	6
IV	2	4	6
Total	10	9	19

Classification of Glasscock and Jackson for Glomus Tumors

I. Small tumour involving the jugular bulb, middle ear and mastoid
II. Tumour extending under internal auditory canal; might have intracranial extension
III. Tumour extending into petrous apex; might have intracranial extension
IV. Tumour extending beyond petrous apex into clivus or infratemporal fossa; might have intracranial extension

Table 2. *Distribution of Tumour Type in 19 Patients with Glomus Jugulare Tumours using the Fisch Classification of Temporal Bone Tumours [18]*

Fisch Subclass	Primary GKRS	Secondary GKRS	Total
C2	2	2	4
C2De1	2	–	2
C2De1Di1	1	1	2
C2De2Di1	–	1	1
C3De1	2	–	2
C3De1Di1	1	2	3
C3De1Di2	1	–	1
C4De1	1	–	1
C4De1Di1	–	2	2
C4De1Di2	–	1	1
Total	10	9	19

Staging Systme of Fisch

A. Limited to mesotympanum
B. Limited to hypotympanum, mesotympanum, and mastoid without erosion of jugular bulb
C. Involvement and destruction of infralabyrinthine and apical compartments.
Subclassification by degree of carotid canal erosion
C1: No invasion of carotid; destruction of jugular bulb/foramen
C2: Invasion of vertical carotid canal between foramen and bend
C3: Invasion along horizontal carotid canal
C4: Invasion of foramen lacerum and along carotid into cavernous sinus
D. Intracranial extension (De, extradural; Di, intradural)
De1: Up to 2-cm dural displacement
De2: More than 2-cm dural displacement
Di1: Up to 2-cm intradural extension
Di2: More than 2-cm intradural extension

Table 3. *Distribution of Pre- and Postradiosurgical Cranial Nerve Deficits and Clinical Symptoms in 19 Patients with Glomus Jugulare Tumours*

Cranial nerve deficit/ clinical symptom	Prior to GKRS no. of patients (%)	Following GKRS no. of patients (%)
Abducent nerve palsy	2 (10.5)	1 (5.3)
Facial nerve palsy	6 (31.6)	4 (21)
Hearing loss	13 (68.4)	13 (68.4)
Tinnitus	10 (52.6)	6 (31.6)
Dysphagia	8 (42.8)	7 (36.8)
Hoarseness	8 (42.8)	6 (31.6)
Accessory nerve palsy	4 (21)	4 (21)
Hypoglossal nerve palsy	5 (26.3)	4 (21)
Ataxia	2 (10.5)	1 (5.3)
Vertigo	4 (21)	3 (15.8)
Cephalea	3 (15.8)	1 (5.3)
Aural haemorrhage	1 (5.3)	0 (0)
Otalgia	2 (10.5)	0 (0)

GKRS. In one patient with an extensive glomus jugulare tumour we performed two-staged radiosurgical treatment to avoid adverse radiation-related tissue effects. The interval between radiosurgical procedures was 6 months. All of the 19 patients had cranial nerve deficits prior to radiosurgery. The distribution of presenting clinical symptoms and signs at the time of GKRS is summarized in Table 3.

An image-compatible Leksell stereotactic coordinate head frame was fixed under local anaesthesia before high-resolution contrast-enhanced CT- or gadolinium-enhanced MRI-based tumour localization. Calibre measurements were carried out in three separate dimensions before and after GKRS. Tumour enlargement or regression was defined as a change of ± 2 mm. Volumetry was calculated at the time of GKRS but not available for all patients in the follow-up as some imaging controls were conducted by peripheral radiologists. At time of GKRS tumour volumes ranged from 0.38 to 33.5 ccm (median 5.22 ccm). Image-integrated treatment planning was performed with the aid of Kula or GammaPlan software. One or more isocentres (range: 1–11, median 5) were used to construct a radiation field suitable to the shape of the tumours. Specific dose selection was guided by tumour volume, history of previous irradiation and proximity of radiosensitive structures. The dose was calculated by determining the tumour volume and the use of the integrated logistic equation for a 3% risk of permanent symptomatic brain injury [8]. The tumour margins received doses of 12 to 20 Gy (median 14 Gy) at the covering isodose line (range 30–55%, median 50%). Maximum tumour doses ranged from 24 to 40 Gy (median 30 Gy). All patients were discharged the day after GKRS and were able to resume their preradiosurgical functional level within 3 to 5 days. Postradiosurgical imaging and clinical controls were requested after 6 months, 12 months and yearly thereafter.

Results

Except for an 81-year-old patient who died 9 months after radiosurgery unrelated to tumour or GKRS, the observation period ranged from 1.5 to 10 years (median 7.2 years). The total tumour control rate was 94.7%. The follow-up imaging studies showed reduced tumour volume in 7 patients (36.8%) and

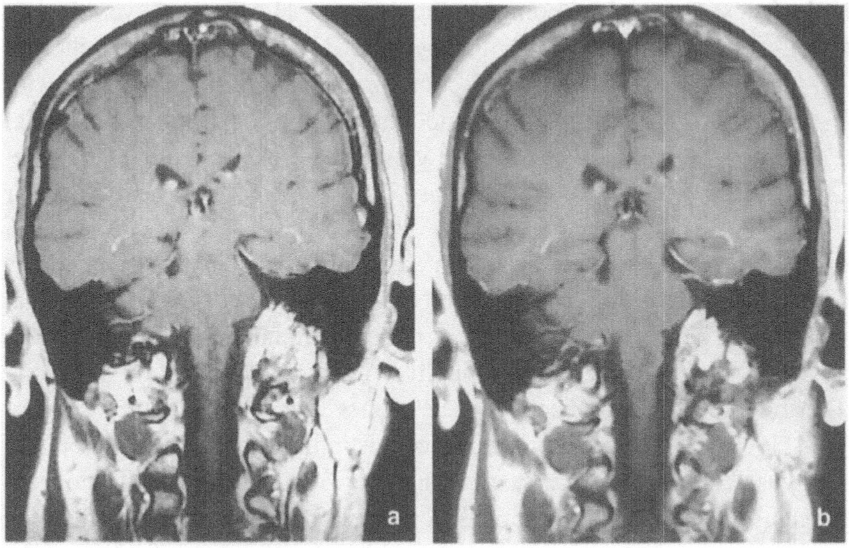

Fig. 1. (a) Planning MRI (gadolinium-enhanced, t1-weighted, coronal view) obtained in a 44-year-old patient with progressive growth of left sided residual paraganglioma 3.8 years after microsurgical resection and conventional radiotherapy. The tumour volume of 13.7 ccm received a marginal dose of 15 Gy at the 50% isodoseline. (b) Recent follow-up scan, performed 101 months after GKRS, displaying local control with unchanged tumour extension, but reduced contrast enhancement in the lower portion of the lesion. Clinically the patient noted normalisation of dysphonia.

unchanged tumour size in 11 cases (57.9%). In one patient (5,3%) the partially resected benign paraganglioma resumed growing 84 months after GKRS. Careful analysis revealed that failure to attain local control was due to undertreatment as it was not possible to define the exact extent of the infrabasal tumour portion on the CT planning scans. Using Kaplan-Meier method the progression free survival rate was calculated 100% for the first seven years and decreased afterwards to 87.5%. Another patient with incompletely removed benign paraganglioma was found with new appearance of a second lesion in the cavernous sinus (5,3%) 52 months after radiosurgical treatment. CT and MRI demonstrated heterogeneous or reduced contrast enhancement in 7 patients (see Fig. 1) and decreased flow voids in 4 cases, but these findings were not related to tumour size (see Table 4).

On clinical examination 10 patients (52,6%) presented with improved and 8 patients (42,1%) with unchanged neurological status. The deterioration in one patient (5,3%) developing 3 months after GKRS during attempted endovascular embolisation for further treatment of persistent tinnitus at a local hospital was not related to tumour or radiosurgery but caused by stroke. The distribution of pre- and postradiosurgical cranial nerve deficits and clinical symptoms is detailed in Table 3.

Four patients received additional treatment for their glomus tumours. Eighty-five months after initial GKRS the only patient with enlarged tumour volume and stable clinical status underwent a second radiosurgical procedure for the portion of the paraganglioma progressing into the clivus. The patient with new appearance of a second lesion at distant site refused open surgery and was treated radiosurgically 53 months after the first Gamma Knife procedure as well. One patient with unchanged clinical status (headache, tinnitus, hearing loss and dizziness) and stable tumour volume requested tumour removal 34 months after primary stereotactic radiosurgery. The surgical intervention, performed by our ENT colleagues, resulted only in partial resection of the tumour, which histologically was classified as benign paraganglioma. The patient with probative endovascular treatment following GKRS was mentioned before. Two patients, aged 81 and 76 years, with un-

Table 4. *Neuroradiological Image Changes following GKRS in 19 Patients with Glomus Jugulare Tumours related to Tumour Size*

Tumour size	Heterogeneous contrast enhancement	Reduced contrast enhancement	Loss of flow voids
Smaller (7 Pts)	2	1	1
Unchanged (11 Pts)	2	1	2
Progressive (1 Pt)	1	–	1

changed tumour volume and stable neurological status died due to unrelated disease at an observation time of 9 and 18 months, respectively.

Discussion

Many authors consider radical resection with preservation of juxtaposed neurovascular structures the therapeutic main stay for paragangliomas of the jugulare foramen [2, 10–12, 20, 24, 27, 28]. Several reports have highlighted the significant morbidity and mortality associated with surgical treatment [4, 14, 19, 22, 25, 26]. In reviewing prior to 1987 published cases, Carrasco *et al.* [3] found tumour persistence in 6%, recurrent growth in 7% and death from tumour progression in 2,5% of the patients after primary surgical treatment. Successful salvage with surgery was observed in 96% of the patients. In the more recent series complete resection of larger glomus jugulare tumours is cited within a range of 41–100%. The postmicrosurgical mortality rate varies from 0% to 4% [1, 2, 10–12, 18, 20, 25, 27, 28]. Postoperative CND was found in up to 76.5%, but in many of the younger patients impaired cranial nerve function was transient or could be rehabilitated to good functional results, whereas elderly patients usually did not recover to a point of useful and enjoyable lives [1, 2, 10–12, 18–20, 25, 27, 28]. Treatment-related complications occurred in 0 to 16.3% of the surgically treated patients [1, 2, 11, 12, 18, 20, 27, 28]. Following surgical resection total rates of local tumour control vary between 90 and 100% [1, 2, 10–12, 18, 20, 25, 28]. Due to the large range of the follow-up periods of the reports on surgical treatment it is difficult to compare the results of the various series [1, 2, 10–12, 18, 20, 25, 27, 28]. Therefore life table or Kaplan-Meier analysis should be applied to determine the rate of tumour control with respect to the length of follow-up as was performed only in one surgical report [27].

The efforts at complete tumour excision should be tempered by patient's age, medical condition, type of neurological deficit, previous surgical treatment and potential risk for unacceptable morbidity or mortality [2, 14, 18, 19, 24, 27]. Comparing patients with surgical and patients without any treatment for glomus jugulare tumours Van der Mey *et al.* [25] noted no difference in survival for the two groups except for surgical-induced morbidity and recommended therefore a more conservative approach, in terms of "wait and see" policy, to these lesions. However, as even the histologically benign, slowly growing paragangliomas have a predilection for local aggressive behaviour with compression and infiltration of adjacent bone, cranial nerves or blood vessels it seems wise to treat these lesions before they involve important neurovascular structures, cause severe neurological deficits or reach larger extension with subsequent higher risk for any treatment option [16, 17]. Sen *et al.* [24] observed that meningiomas or paragangliomas of the jugulare foramen tend to infiltrate the cranial nerves IX–XI along connective tissue planes due to their multifascicular architecture. Since this infiltration may be present despite normal cranial nerve function radical tumour removal implies a high risk for severe disability and may sometimes not be achieved without sacrification of the involved cranial nerves [2, 24].

In patients with residual or recurrent tumours despite microsurgical resection or considerable associated disease alternative strategies should be used [1, 2, 11, 12, 14, 19, 20, 27, 28].

Carrasco *et al.* [3] reviewed 24 series, reported between 1964 and 1987, to define the value of radiation therapy for glomus jugulare tumours. Following primary radiotherapy 11% of the patients had persistent paragangliomas, tumour recurrence occurred in 8% of the cases and 6% of the patients died from the disease. Radiation salvage was successful in 86% of the patients.

Other reports on radiotherapeutic treatment for jugulare foramen paragangliomas related that tumour control could be obtained in 88%–100% of the patients [4, 14, 22, 26]. Postirradiation complications developed in up to 5.3% of the patients, but as many series did not detail exact information the absolute complication rate might be much higher. Death from uncontrollable tumour progression was cited in 0 to 10.5% of the patients following radiation therapy and lethal radiation-induced encephalopathy was seen as well [4, 14, 22, 26].

Endovascular occlusion of feeding vessels may be performed as a complementary treatment measure to reduce the tumoural vascular supply before surgical resection and prior to radiotherapy or stereotactic radiosurgery [1, 6, 9, 13, 15, 17, 18, 20, 21, 27]. On the basis of their experience with the histopathological sections in 35 preoperatively embolized paragangliomas of stage C and D Pauw *et al.* [21], recommended to operate within 8 days after embolisation. They observed that only one third of the tumour vessels were occluded using polyvinyl alcohol as embolic agent. After 9 to 16 days partial revascularization involved 30% of the embolized vessels and complete obliteration occurred in 40% of the embolized vessels more than 2 months following selective embolisation. Therefore embolisation alone cannot guarantee complete devitalisation of paragangliomas and has to be considered a palliative treatment option [20].

Within the last years, only a few publications mentioned the application of GKRS as non-invasive alternative therapeutic modality for patients who are poor candidates for surgery and as adjuvant treatment option for subtotally resected tumours or recurrences after surgical interventions, as well [5, 6, 9, 13, 15–17, 23]. GKRS is designed to accurately deliver a single high dose of stereotactically focused gamma radiation to an intracranial target. The steep dose gradient achievable with this technique guarantees maximum sparing of surrounding normal tissue [9, 13, 16, 17, 23]. Since glomus jugulare tumours are usually highly vascularized, well circumscribed and easily delineated on radiographic findings they are ideally suited for GKRS [23]. In our current series we included the results of our previously published reports on radiosurgical treatment of large glomus jugulare tumours [5, 6, 15] with smaller patient numbers and shorter observation periods. After up to 10 years follow-up local tumour control was achieved in 18 of 19 patients (94,7%) following GKRS. Reduction in tumour size was observed in 36.8% of the patients. Failure to achieve local control in one patient (5.3%) was caused by incomplete treatment, as the CT planning scans did not clearly display the infrabasal tumour extent. Ten patients (52,6%) remained clinically unchanged whereas 8 patients (42.1%) experienced permanent improvement or normalization of neurological disorders due to recovery of cranial nerve function or reduced brain-stem compression. Clinical deterioration developing only in one patient was not related to GKRS or tumour and no complication occurred.

After an observation time of 7–65 months (median 20 months) Foote *et al.* [9] reported local tumour control in all of the 9 patients (100%) treated with the gamma knife for glomus tumours. Tumour size was reduced in one patient (11%) and remained stable in 8 patients (89%). Neurological status was unaltered in 2 patients (22%), while 7 patients (78%) noted clinical amelioration. Consistent with our own observations they found no complication or treatment-related side effects.

Following GKRS Liščák *et al.* [16] observed no progressive growth in 14 patients with glomus jugulare tumours at a median observation period of 20.5 months (range from 6 to 42 months). Tumour size was decreased in 4 patients and unchanged in the remaining cases. Six patients experienced clinical improvement and preservation of cranial nerve function was achieved in all but 3 cases with further hearing deterioration on the affected side.

Jordan *et al.* [13], related tumour control in all of the 7 patients (3 cases with unaltered and 4 cases with reduced tumour volume) available for neuroradiological follow-up after GKRS. One out of 8 patients developed acute onset of intractable vertigo with increased dysequilibrium subsiding only during the following 11 months. After an average observation time of 27 months (range: 7–102 months) 3 patients were found with improved tinnitus, two with ameliorated hearing, one with decreased vertigo and another patient with decreased deglutition difficulties.

Recently, Saringer *et al.* [23] published their experience with GKRS in the treatment of glomus jugulare tumours in 13 patients with an observation period of up to 6.7 years. They observed decreased tumour size in 3 and stable tumour volume in 10 patients. Clinically 6 patients remained unchanged, 6 patients improved and one patient was lost to follow-up. Two patients developed transient radiation induced complications (worsening of pre-existent swallowing disorders and temporary facial nerve palsy) 1 and 12 months after radiosurgical treatment, respectively.

As all Gamma Knife series comprise only a small number of cases a multicentre study was performed collecting the data from 6 European institutions [17]. After an average follow-up time of 24 months (range 4 to 70 months) no progression was found in the 47 patients with available follow-up scans. Tumour size was unaltered in 28 patients (60%) and reduced in 19 patients (40%). Fifteen out of 52 patients (29%) experienced clinical amelioration. Five patients were found with deteriorated neurological status, but worsening was unrelated to tumour or GKRS in two cases and transient (impaired tinnitus) in another patient. At 24 months after GKRS pre-existent facial nerve palsy and decreased hearing worsened permanently in one patient and further impairment of facial nerve function and aggravated vertigo developed 6 months after GKRS in the second patient with persisting morbidity.

Feigenberg *et al.* [7] reported local control in 3 out of 5 temporal bone paragangliomas with a follow-up period of 14 to 50 months (median 27 months) following Linac-based stereotactic radiosurgery. The 2 patients with progressive growth showed clinical deterioration, while the remaining patients were found with stable or improved symptoms. Their results are apparently worse than those reported after GKRS.

After successful GKRS of paragangliomas heterogeneous or reduced contrast enhancement is the exception and not the rule on CT or MRI follow-up studies [15, 16, 23]. Complete disappearance or reduction of pathological vascularisation may be found on postradiosurgical control angiographies, but these changes are no indicator for local tumour control or treatment success [16, 17]. Endovascular embolisation before or after GKRS can result in considerable morbidity. Thus, this procedure should be carried out only when the expected benefit balances its potential risks and has to be performed by experienced interventional radiologists [6, 17]. It is difficult to prove that clinical amelioration is due to GKRS as even postoperative impaired cranial nerve function may recover with time [2, 19]. Nevertheless treatment-related morbidity after GKRS, if present, is generally very low and usually transient and compares favourably with the results of the other treatment options [1, 2, 4–7, 9–20, 22, 23, 25–28].

Conclusion

As physicians it is our continuing goal to select the optimum therapeutic strategy for the individual patient, in terms of disease control and maintenance of quality of life. Treatment options for glomus jugulare tumours comprise surgery, radiotherapy, radiosurgery or observation only. The decision should be made in accordance with the patient on the basis of patient's age, general medical condition, degree of neurological impairment, tumour size and growth rate, previous therapy and potential risk for treatment-related morbidity or mortality. In younger patients or cases with brain stem compression surgical resection with preservation of major vessels and cranial nerves should be performed as primary treatment but the degree of resection should be limited to partial removal rather than radical resection to avoid additional clinical deterioration. As the results following GKRS are better than those achieved with conventional radiotherapy or Linac-based radiosurgery recurrent or residual glomus tumours should be treated with GKRS. In patients with considerable associated disease, advanced age or high risk for severe postoperative disability or individuals who refuse surgical treatment GKRS has to be considered as primary alternative therapy.

However, due to the long natural history of jugulare foramen paragangliomas observation periods from at least 10 to 20 years are required before any final conclusion regarding the various treatment options can be expected.

References

1. Anand VK, Leonetti JP and Al-Mefty O (1993) Neurovascular considerations in surgery of glomus tumors with intracranial extensions. Laryngoscope 103 [Suppl] 60: 722–728
2. Briner HR, Linder TE, Pauw B, Fisch U (1999) Long-term results of surgery for temporal bone paragangliomas. Laryngoscope 109: 577–583
3. Carrasco V and Rosenman J (1993) Radiation therapy of glomus jugulare tumors. Laryngoscope 103 [Suppl] 60: 23–27
4. Cole JM and Beiler D (1994) Long-term results of treatment for glomus jugulare and glomus vagale tumors with radiotherapy. Laryngoscope 104: 1461–1465
5. Eustacchio S, Trummer M, Unger F, Schröttner O, Papaefthymiou G, Feichtinger K, Pendl G (1998) Stereotaktische radiochirurgische Behandlung von Glomustumoren. In: Lanksch WR, Lehmann ThN (eds) Die hintere Schädelgrube und der kraniozervikale Übergang. Reinbek, Einhorn Presse Verlag, pp 153–157
6. Eustacchio S, Leber K, Trummer M, Unger F, Pendl G (1999) Gamma knife radiosurgery for glomus jugulare tumours. Acta Neurochir (Wien) 141: 811–818
7. Feigenberg SJ, Mendenhall WM, Hinerman RW, Amdur RJ, Friedman WA, Antonelli PJ (2002) Radiosurgery for paraganglioma of the temporal bone. Head Neck 24: 384–389
8. Flickinger JC (1989) An integrated logistic formula for prediction of complications from radiosurgery. Int J Radiat Oncol Biol Phys 17: 879–885
9. Foote RL, Coffey RJ, Gorman DA, Earle JD, Schomberg PJ, Kline RW and Schild SE (1997) Stereotactic radiosurgery for glomus jugulare tumors: a preliminary report. Int J Radiat Oncol Biol Phys 38: 491–495
10. George B and Huy PTB (2000) Surgical resection of jugulare foramen tumours by juxtacondylar approach without facial nerve transposition. Acta Neurochir (Wien) 142: 613–620
11. Gjuric M, Seidinger L and Wigand ME (1996) Long-term results of surgery for temporal bone paraganglioma. Skull base surgery 6: 147–152
12. Green JD, Brackmann DE, Nguyen CD, Arriaga MA, Telischi FF and De la Cruz A (1994) Surgical management of previously untreated glomus jugulare tumors. Laryngoscope 104: 917–921
13. Jordan JA, Roland PS, McManus C, Weiner RL, Giller CA (2000) Stereotactic radiosurgery for glomus jugulare tumors. Laryngoscope 110: 35–38
14. Larner JM, Hahn SS, Spaulding CA and Constable WC (1992) Glomus jugulare tumors. Long-term control by radiation therapy. Cancer 69: 1813–1817
15. Leber KA, Eustacchio S, Pendl G (1999) Radiosurgery of glomus tumors: midterm results. Stereotact Funct Neurosurg 72 [Suppl] 1: 53–59
16. Liščák R, Vladyka V, Šimonová G, Vymazal J, Janoušková L (1998) Leksell gamma knife radiosurgery of the tumour glomus

jugulare and tympanicum. Stereotact Funct Neurosurg 70 [Suppl] 1: 152–160
17. Liščák R, Vladyka V, Wowra B, Kemeny A, Forster D, Burzaco JA, Martinez R, Eustacchio S, Pendl G, Regis J, Pellet W (1999) Gamma Knife radiosurgery of the glomus jugulare tumour – early multicentre experience. Acta Neurochir (Wien) 141: 1141–1146
18. Moe KS, Li D, Linder TE, Schmid S, and Fisch U (1999) An update on the surgical treatment of temporal bone paraganglioma. Skull base surgery 9: 185–194
19. Netterville JL, Civantos FJ (1993) Rehabilitation of cranial nerve deficits after neurotologic skull base surgery. Laryngoscope 103 [Suppl] 60: 45–54
20. Patel SJ, Sekhar LN, Cass SP and Hirsch BE (1994) Combined approaches for resection of extensive glomus jugulare tumors: a review of 12 cases. J Neurosurg 80: 1026–1038
21. Pauw BK, Makek MS, Fisch U and Valvanis A (1993) Preoperative embolisation of paragangliomas (glomus tumors) of the head and neck: histopathologic and clinical features. Skull base surgery 3: 37–44
22. Powell S, Peters N and Harmer C (1992) Chemodectoma of the head and neck: results of treatment in 84 patients. Int J Radiat Oncol Biol Phys 22: 919–924
23. Saringer W, Khayal H, Ertl A, Schoeggl A, Kitz-K (2001) Efficiency of gamma knife radiosurgery in the treatment of glomus jugulare tumors. Minim Invas Neurosurg 44: 141–145
24. Sen C, Hague K, Kacchara,R, Jenkins A, Das S, Catalano P (2001) Jugular foramen: microscopic anatomic features and implications for neural preservation with reference to glomus tumors involving the temporal bone. Neurosurgery 48: 838–847
25. Van der Mey AGL, Frijns JHM, Cornelisse CJ, Brons EN, Van Dulken H, Terpstra HL, Schmidt PH (1992) Does intervention improve the natural course of glomus tumors? A series of 108 patients seen in a 32-year period. Ann Otol Rhinol Laryngol 101: 635–642
26. Wang ML, Hussey DH, Doornbos JF, Vigliotti AP and Wen BC (1988) Chemodectoma of the temporal bone: a comparison of surgical and radiotherapeutic results. Int J Radiat Oncol Biol Phys 14: 643–648
27. Watkins LD, Mendoza N, Cheesman AD, Symon L (1994) Glomus jugulare tumours: a review of 61 cases. Acta Neurochir (Wien) 130: 66–70
28. Woods CI, Strasnick B and Jackson CG (1993) Surgery for glomus tumors: the otolgy group experience. Laryngoscope 103 [Suppl] 60: 65–70

Correspondence: Dr. Sandro Eustacchio, Department of Neurosurgery, Karl-Franzens University, Auenbruggerplatz 29, 8036 Graz, Austria.

Acta Neurochir (2002) [Suppl] 84: 99–105

Radiation and Regeneration: Behavioral Improvement and GDNF Expression after Gamma Knife Radiosurgery in the 6-OHDA Rodent Model of Hemi-Parkinsonism

V. A. Zerris, Z. Zheng, G. Noren, A. Sungarian, and **G. M. Friehs**

Department of Clinical Neurosciences (Neurosurgery) and New England Gamma Knife Center, Brown University, Providence, Rhode Island, USA

Summary

Background. Recent research has demostrated that the adult mammalian CNS is capable of regeneration. This regeneration is often initiated as a response to thermal, chemical or mechanical injury. The effects of radiation on the mammalian CNS have also been found to aid in certain regeneration processes.

Method. In our project we examined the potential therapeutic value of radiation induced regeneration of diseased mammalian rat CNS. Eleven Sprague-Dawley rats with 6-hydroxy-dopamine (6-OHDA) induced hemi-parkinsonism were treated in the Leksell Gamma Knife using a single 4 mm collimator shot targeted to the ipsilateral (parkinsonian) caudate-putamen complex. A maximum dose of 140 Gy was used to create a necrotic lesion. Animals were tested behaviorally using the apomorphine-induced rotational behavior model before and up to 6 months after radiosurgery. Histochemical analysis was performed 2 weeks, 1 month and 4 months after radiosurgery. Histological sections were obtained and immunohistochemistry was performed for glial cell line derived neurotrophic factor (GDNF).

Findings. The rotational behavior for 11/11 animals (100%) was found to initially worsen at 2 weeks and 4 weeks after radiosurgery before a statistically highly significant reduction in apomorphine induced rotations was observed at 2, 3, and 4 months after radiosurgery (83% reduction by month four; $p < 0.0001$). For 2/11 animals the rotational behavior almost disappeared indicating near-abolition of parkinsonian behavior. On histological examination, the lesions were easily identified as areas of necrosis about 4 mm in diameter. The region immediately adjacent to the lesion was found to have highly positive expression of GDNF indicating high activity in dopamine-regenerating processes.

Interpretation. In this preliminary study we demonstrated that radiosurgical lesioning with the Gamma Knife into the striatum of hemi-parkinsonian animals resulted in significant behavioral improvement of signs of parkinsonism. Since GDNF expression is tightly linked to the dopaminergic system, we conclude that focused radiation is potentially capable of inducing regeneration of dopaminergic pathways in the adult CNS. Further studies with dose de-escalation and molecular biological characterization of the regeneration cascades are necessary to gain access to potential clinical value of our observations.

Keywords: Radiosurgery; regeneration; parkinsonism; neurotrophic factors.

Introduction

Parkinsonism is characterized by a loss of dopaminergic projections between the Substantia Nigra (SN) and the striatum. The mainstay of treatment is focused on replacement therapy by administering dopamine precursors or analogs as oral drugs. It has become apparent that long-term drug therapy induces tolerance and is associated with severe side effects that are often as disabling as the disease itself. Therefore, over the past 20 years, intensive research has been conducted to find new therapeutic regimens. Transplantation neurosurgery was believed to be a promising approach. Grafting dopaminergic tissue into the diseased dopamine-depleted parkinsonian striatum was thought to restore function by providing a living source of the missing transmitter inside the CNS. Neuro-transplantation, especially with fetal tissue, has raised serious ethical concerns [7, 16, 19–21, 26]. Strong evidence has accumulated that grafting of dopaminergic tissue might not even be the only factor responsible for the restoration of lost function. In one of our own studies using the 6-hydroxy-dopamine (6-OHDA) model of hemiparkinsonian rats, we showed in a controlled trial that lesioning of the striatum is significantly more effective than transplanting dopaminergic tissue and leads to near abolition of parkinsonian behavior in the rat. Shortly after, a controlled trial was designed with four groups of hemiparkinsonian rats [13]. Group I only received 6-OHDA lesions of the SN, thus serving as the control. Group II comprised 6-OHDA treated rats that reveived autologous adrenal medullary grafts into the caudate-putamen complex. The third group was comprised of 6-OHDA rats that received thermal radiofrequency lesions in the striatum ipsilateral to the 6-OHDA lesion. Group IV included 6-OHDA rats that received grafts into a cavity created by previous radiofrequency lesioning in an attempt to enhance graft survival. Behavioral assessment was undertaken using the rotational rat model with injection of apomorphine, a direct dopamine agonist. It was found that the groups receiving grafts showed a reduction in rotational behavior which was significant when compared to the controls. However, the two groups receiving radiofrequency-lesions of the striatum demonstrated an even more significant amelioration of symptoms when compared to the control animals and the grafted animals. Immunohistochemical analysis of these animals revealed a dense area of tyrosine-hydroxylase positive fibers adjacent to the lesions within the otherwise dopamine-depleted striatum, therefore causing partial reinnervation of the striatum.

Plunkett, Bankiewicz and coauthors reported dramatic improvement in the MPTP primate model of hemiparkinsonism after transplantation or the creation of a cavity in the striatum [2–5, 23, 25]. They also showed that even if transplanted tissue did not survive, there was still significant behavioral improvement. This is further underlined by post-mortem analyses in human studies [9–10, 22, 28]. The origin of these regenerating fibers was speculated to be in the nucleus accumbens and the area olfactoria [23]. Based on our own experience and strongly supported by the above mentioned reports, a clinical trial was designed and carried out [11–12]. Nine patients with severe bradykinesia-dominant parkinsonism were enrolled in the study and bilateral lesioning of the Caudate Nucleus (CN) was performed with the Gamma Knife. After an observation period ranging from one to twelve months, a beneficial effect was found in 90% of the patients. When taken as a group and compared to preoperative values, there was significant improvement of motor function one month after treatment. Since there were no complications associated with this type of treatment, histological or immunohistochemical data was not available. In search for possible mechanisms underlying these findings the role of growth factor mediated neuronal regeneration has been proposed. Special interest has been focused on Glial Derived Neurotrophic Factor which specifically promotes the survival of dopaminergic neurons. GDNF was isolated in 1993, and is a glycosylated, dysulfied bonded, homodimer that is structurally related to the transforming growth factor-beta superfamily [18]. A number of functions and targets have been described for GDNF. In vivo studies of lesioned animals include both mechanical and chemical lesions. When dopaminergic neurons were induced to degenerate by transecting the axons in the medial forebrain bundle, GDNF injections next to the substantia nigra prevented this loss [6]. A number of studies have been performed in order to assess GDNF's ability to prevent neurotoxins from causing the degeneration of dopamine neurons. In addition some researches have focused on the ability of GDNF to reverse the effects of neurotoxins. A single administration of GDNF into 6-OHDA lesioned animals was able to significantly reduce the apomorphine induced rotational behavior [14], which measures the extent of the lesion produced by 6-OHDA and is inversely proportional to dopamine levels [15]. In another study, the animals were given a series of four injections on days 1, 3, 5 and 8 post lesion. A range of different doses were used, including 0.1, 1, and 10 micrograms. Once more, the treatment significantly reduced the development of amphetamine induced rotations [24]. In a controlled study it was shown that GDNF pretreated rats showed almost 5 times the survival rate of dopamine neurons when exposed to 6-OHDA compared to PBS pretreated rats (49% Vs 9%) [17]. Grafting of genetically engineered fibroblasts expressing high levels of GDNF has been shown to prevent more than 80% of the 6-OHDA induced degeneration of noradrenergic neurons in the locus coeruleus [1]. These results have been reproduced by a number of other researchers. GDNF has been shown to be protective against a number of other neurotoxins. GDNF injected over the substantia nigra or in the striatum before 1-methyl-4-phenyl-1,2,3,6-tetrahydropyridine treatment potently protects the dopaminergic system [27]. GDNF also selectively protects dopamine neurons over 5-HT neurons against methamphetamine toxicity [8]. In summary, our preliminary studies furnish evidence for regenerative potential of the diseased adult mammalian CNS on the cellular level as well as the functional outcome level. The purpose of this experiment was to determine whether a Gamma Knife lesion on the ipsilateral side of unilateral 6-OHDA treated rats would lead to an upregulation of GDNF expression around the lesion, and whether this would correlate with a decrease in apomorphine induced rotational behavior.

Materials and Methods

Adult male Sprague-Dawley rats weighing 250–300 g were used for our experiments. Animals were purchased after the 6-OHDA injection was performed and the effects of unilateral dopaminergic loss was confirmed (Zivic-Miller). All animals underwent apomorphine induced rotational behavior testing twice to establish a baseline and verify the effectiveness of the unilateral 6-OHDA lesion. Rats whose ipsilateral rotational average did not exceed 200 rotations per hour were excluded Qualifying animals were treated with striatal Gamma Knife ipsilateral to the 6-OHDA lesion. Following Gamma Knife treatment the animals underwent behavioral testing at regular intervals until they were euthanized. Three rats were euthanized one week after radiosurgery for immunohistochemistry, two animals at one month, and six animals at four months after Gamma Knife treatment. In order to control for accuracy and effectiveness of Gamma Knife treatment, animals not showing any signs of lesioning or with a lesion in the wrong anatomical position were excluded. This left a total of eleven rats included in our experiments. Animal health and well being was monitored throughout the duration of the experiment by the Rhode Island Hospital Central Research Laboratories veterinarian.

Gamma Knife Procedure

Standard Gamma Knife procedures similar to the ones for human patients were followed. The animals were first injected with 1 cc/kg of anesthetic solution (Ketamine 25 mg/cc, Xylazine 1.25 mg/cc, Acepromazine 0.25 mg/cc). The effectiveness of anesthesia and analgesia was verified by pinching the animals' paw and tail. The animals were placed and secured in a custom made rodent stereotactic frame adapter. Treatment time and coordinates were calculated using the Gamma Knife computer work station. The maximum dose was 140 Gy using a single 4 mm collimator shot. After completion of treatment the animals were removed from the frame and allowed to regain consciousness. They were then returned to their cages and monitored for possible treatment side effects.

Behavioral Testing

The hardware used in this experiment was the Photobeam Activity Rotometer System® (San Diego Instruments, San Diego, CA). This system includes an 18-inch "pebble-grained" clear acrylic enclosure, an animal band and light spring steel harness with velcro attachments, a photobeam sensory unit, a single chip computer acting as an interface between the rotometer heads and the host computer, and a PC compatible computer with related software, which allowed "real-time" presentation and long term storing of the data.

The rubber band with the velcro loop (chest harness) was placed behind the animal's head and forepaws and attached to the photobeam sensor unit. The animal was placed in the geometric center of the enclosure. Because of its spherical shape, the animal was able to move around comfortably without pulling on the attachment wire. The animal was allowed to acclimate for approximately 10 min. An injection of apomorphine (0.05 mg/kg) was administered intramuscularly. The number of clockwise and counterclockwise rotations was counted and stored on the computer for a total of one hour per testing session. The animal was then removed from the enclosure and returned to its cage after removal of the chest harness.

Immunohistochemistry

Animals were deeply anesthetized using intraperitoneal pentobarbital sodium (50 mg/kg). They were then transcardially perfused with 100 ml of pre-chilled (~4 °C) heparinized (25 IU/ml) 0.9% NaCl solution. This was followed by 250 ml of pre-chilled 4% paraformaldehyde in 0.05 M phosphate buffered saline (PBS, pH 7.4). Animals were then decapitated. Using blunt dissection the cranial cavity was opened and the entire cerebrum and cerebellum were carefully removed. The tissue was then post-fixed for 2 hours at 4 °C in paraformaldehyde solution and was incubated in 20% sucrose (0.05 M PBS) at 4 °C for 12 hours.

The cerebellum and the posterior 6 millimeters of the cerebrum were removed. Each brain was then positioned anterior-end down in a labeled polypropylene embedding mold (Polysciences, Inc, Warrington, PA) containing Tissue Tek® O.C.T. Compound (Scientific Products, Boston, MA) and additional O.C.T. compound was added, sufficient to cover the tissue. The embedding mold was floated on the surface of liquid nitrogen until the tissue and surrounding O.C.T. compound were frozen (approximately 15 sec.) Frozen specimens were left in the embedding molds and transferred immediately to a deep freezer for storage overnight.

The next day the frozen specimens were removed from the −80 °C freezer, placed in the cryostat (Reichert-Jung Cryocut 1800) and allowed to warm to cryostat cabinet temperature (−22 °C). Frozen sections were cut at a thickness of 10 microns, picked up on room temperature Superfrost Plus glass microscope slides (Fisher Scientific, Springfield, NJ) and placed into pre-chilled microscope slide boxes in the cryostat chamber until sectioning was complete. Slide boxes were then closed in the cryostat chamber and immediately moved to a −80 °C freezer for storage overnight.

The following day, the slides were first allowed to thaw for approximately 15 min at room temperature. They were then placed in Saponin buffer (10 μg/ml) for 30 min. They were quenched for 5 min in a solution made of 25 ml of 30% H_2O_2 and 225 ml of MeOH. They were rinsed with tap water for 5 min. Proteinase K (Boeringer Mannheim, Germany) was added for 5 min. They were washed in Saponin buffer three times over a 15 min period. The endogenous biotin was then blocked, using an Avidin/Biotin Blocking Kit (Vector Laboratories, Burlingame, CA.) The kit contained avidin and biotin which were diluted 1 : 20 with carrier solution. The slides were first incubated in diluted avidin solution and then in diluted biotin solution for 30 min each, with two 10 min washes with Saponin buffer following each incubation. The slides then underwent a normal serum block by being placed in 20% normal goat serum (Sigma). They were then incubated with the rabbit primary antibody at 1 : 100, 1 : 500, 1 : 750 and 1 : 1000 dilutions with 10% NGS and then stored overnight at 4 °C. The next day they were allowed to thaw at room temperature for about 1 hour. They were rinsed in Saponin buffer six times 10 min each for a total of 60 min. Sections were then incubated with secondary anti-rabbit antibody for 1 h (1 : 200 with 0.5% bovine serum albumin). They were washed with Saponin buffer 4 times, 10 min each, for a total of 40 min. They were incubated for one hour at room temperature with streptavidin-biotin-peroxidase-complex (20× concentrated, Vector Laboratories). They were then placed in NaAc (0.1 M) twice for 10 min each, for a total of 20 min. To visualize the immunohistochemical complex they were incubated for 10 min in a solution of 3,3-diaminobenzidinetetrahydrochloride (0 Sigma Chemical Co, St Louis, MO.) Slides were then washed in tap water for 5 min. They were counterstained with methyl green. They were then dehydrated (70% ethanol, 95% ethanol, 100% ethanol, xylene) and coverslipped.

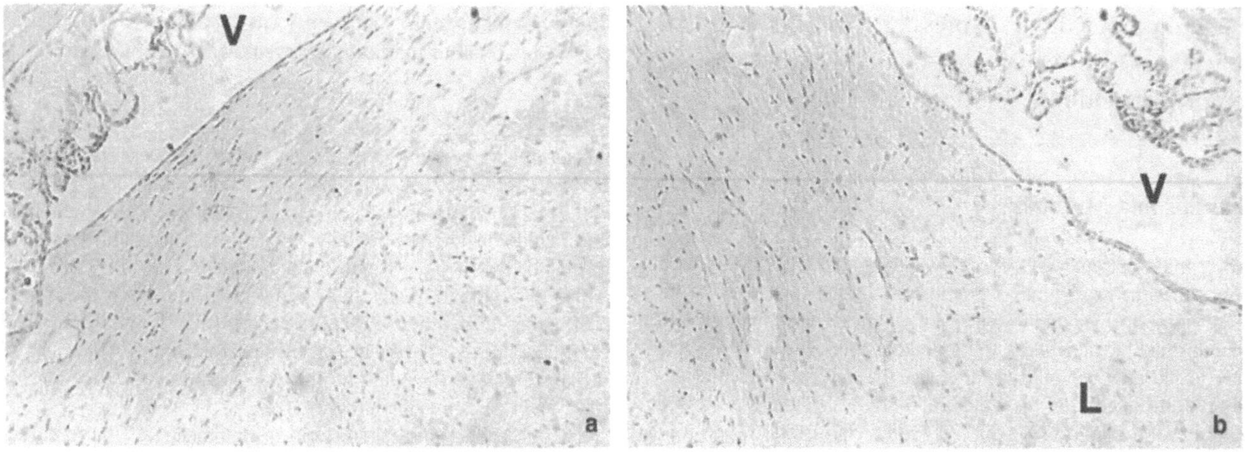

Fig. 1. Low power photomicrograph of rat striatum 1 week after Gamma Knife treatment; GDNF immunohistochemistry, DAB staining, methyl green counterstain. The untreated, non-parkinsonian striatum (a) and the parkinsonian striatum (b) show no significant staining for GDNF. *V* Ventricle; *L* Gamma Knife lesion. Magnification: 200×

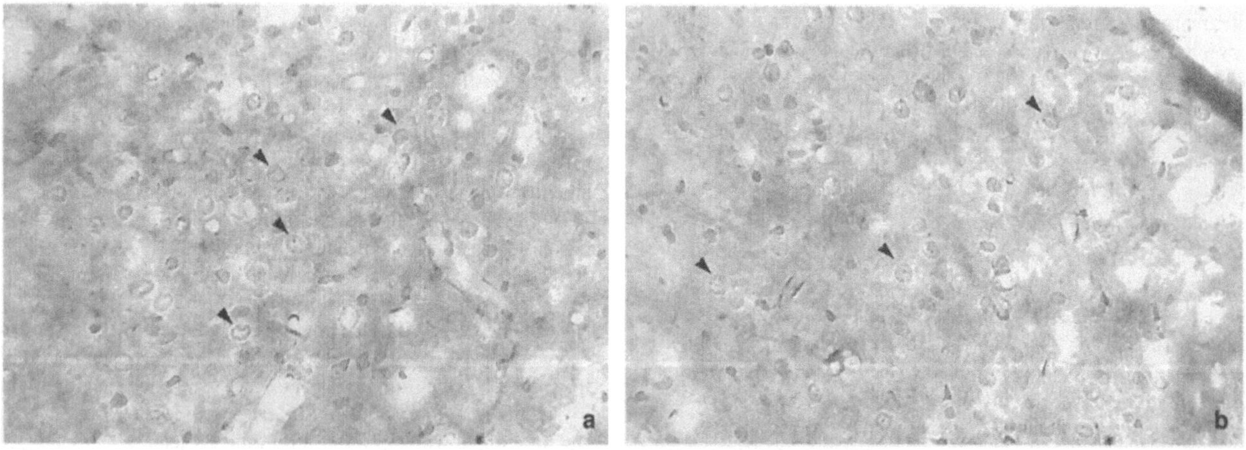

Fig. 2. Medium power photomicrograph of rat striatum 1 month after Gamma Knife treatment; GDNF immunohistochemistry, DAB staininig, methyl green counterstain. Only few cells show some positive GDNF staining. GDNF negative glial cells are marked with arrowheads. Again, there is no significant difference between the untreated side (a) and the radiosurgically treated parkinsonian side (b) Magnification: 400×

Results

Immunohistochemistry

Sections were examined under light microscopy with specific focus to the area adjacent to the Gamma Knife lesion and the corresponding region on the contralateral side of the brain. One week after Gamma Knife treatment neither side showed any significant positive staining for GDNF. One or two cells showed positive staining per high power field in the area of the striatum per section, the number slightly varying from animal to animal (Fig. 1a and 1b).

The one-month group also showed very few positive staining cells. The number of GDNF positive cells was similar to the one week group. Overall staining was negative in both hemispheres (Fig. 2a and 2b).

In the four month group, substantial differences were noted between the treated and untreated sides. The side contralateral to the Gamma Knife lesion showed no significant staining for GDNF (Fig. 3a). The neurons and glia cells on this side stained similar to the background. On the other hand, the area around the Gamma Knife lesion showed significant positive GDNF staining (Fig. 3b). Strongly immunopositive neurons and glia cells were distributed throughout this area. Both cell bodies and processes showed significant staining. There was a significant difference in the number of cells staining and the intensity of the staining between the ipsilateral and contralateral sides.

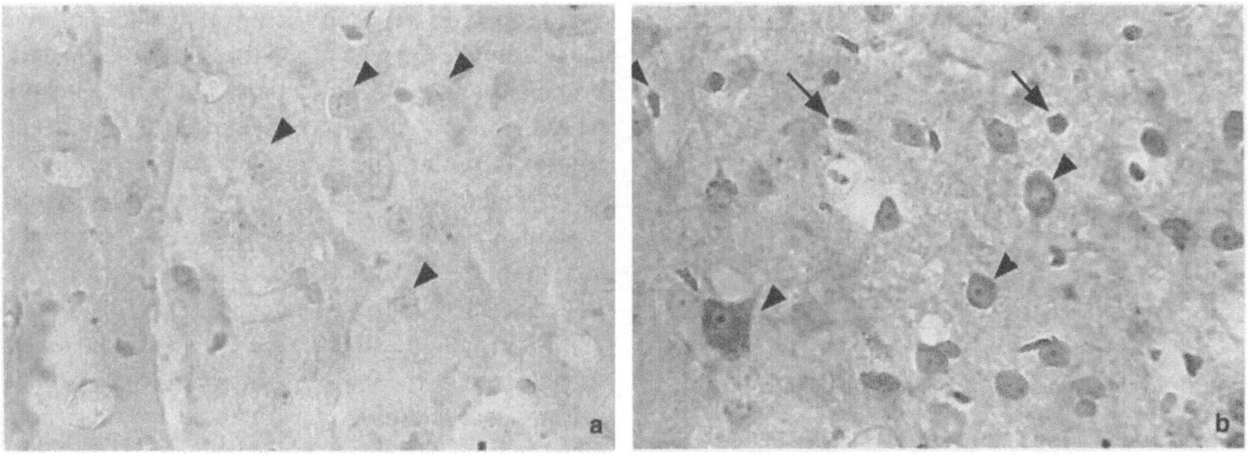

Fig. 3. High power photomicrograph of rat striatum 4 months after Gamma Knife treatment; GDNF immunohistochemistry, DAB staininig, methyl green counterstain. On the untreated side glial cells can be seen which are not stained for GDNF (a) arrowheads. In the 6-OHDA treated side (b) which received 140 Gy of radiation, there are multiple densely GDNF-positive glial cells and neurons (arrows). Also, cell processes appear to be GDNF positive. Magnification: 800×

In summary, the one week and one month groups showed negative staining for GDNF. Corresponding brain regions on both sides of the brain showed similar morphology and staining patterns for GDNF. In the four month group there is a clear difference in immunoreactivity between the two sides. The untreated side showed negative staining while the lesioned side showed strong positive GDNF staining. Overall, there was an increase over time in positive staining for GDNF around the Gamma Knife lesion while the contralateral side remained grossly negative throughout.

Table 1. *Number of Contralateral Turns per Hour During Apomorphine-Induced Rotational Behavior Testing. Baseline Data is Shown as Average of 2 or more Trials*

Animal	Baseline	1 w post	1 m post	2 m post	3 m post	4 m post
1	257	400	493	62	69	23
2	272	274	448	191	350	90
3	378	504	506	231	84	101
4	255	428	226	112	2	15
5	370	432	302	139	85	85
6	353	509	–	20	12	9
7	238	353	488			
8	261	339	327			
9	297	263				
10	297	343				
11	232	390				

Behavioral Data

When challenged with apomorphine the animals exhibited the typical biphasic rotational pattern. The baseline behavior varied among subjects, but all the rats showed very similar temporal trends. There was an increase in rotations in the first week post Gamma Knife treatment which continued in most of the animals throughout the first month. In the second, third, and fourth months the rotations were significantly reduced. With the exception of one rat, rotations had dropped below the baseline by the second month. By month four, all of the rats showed considerably reduced rotational behavior in comparison to their pre-Gamma Knife values. The data values are presented in Table 1. The initial baseline average for the whole group was 292 rotations/hour. In the first week it increased to 385 rotations/hour and by the first month had reached 413 rotations/hour. In the second, third, and fourth month the average rotations were reduced to 125, 100 and 53 rotations/hour, respectively.

Using a Student's t-test, all observed changes were statistically significant. With the pre-Gamma Knife rotational averages as baseline, the rotational behavior increased significantly one week after treatment ($p < 0.001$) and one month after treatment ($p < 0.005$). Two months after radiosurgery there was a significant reduction in rotational behavior ($p < 0.0001$) which was maintained at three months ($p < 0.0005$) and four months post Gamma Knife treatment ($p < 10^{-7}$).

In the first week post treatment the average increase in rotations was 33.5%. By the first month the rota-

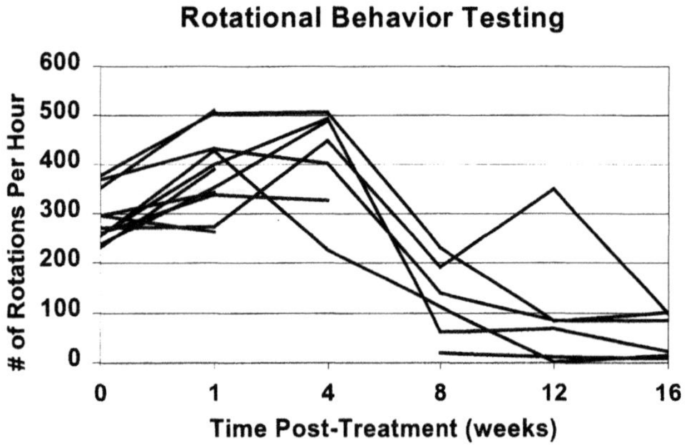

Fig. 4

tions continued to increase, reaching values which were on average 45% higher than the baseline. By the second month the subjects exhibited considerable behavioral improvement with an average decrease in rotations of 59.5% from baseline. This continued into months three and four, the average decrease from baseline reaching 66% and 83% accordingly. These trends are graphically depicted in Fig. 4.

Discussion

In this study, eleven 6-OHDA hemiparkinsonian rats received Gamma Knife treatment at a dose of 140 Gy in the area of the striatum, ipsilateral to the neurotoxin injection. The animals showed consistent behavioral and immunohistochemical effects to the Gamma Knife treatment. There was an increase of rotational behavior in the first month which was followed by a decrease in the next three months. By the fourth month the rotational values were, on average, 83% lower than the pretreatment values. In addition, the rats euthanized at four months showed an upregulation of GDNF expression, which was localized around the area of the Gamma Knife lesion. Both neurons and glia cells stained positively for GDNF.

The correlation between the absence in GDNF and absence of behavioral improvement in the one week and one month group, and the reduction in rotations and increase in GDNF staining in the four month group are consistent with the literature. Exogenously administered GDNF in the rat brain has been shown to reduce apomorphine induced rotations [14]. GDNF has demonstrated the ability to significantly increase the number of TH positive neurons in the substantia nigra of 6-OHDA rats [17]. A number of theories have been proposed to explain these findings. Radioactive injury from the Gamma Knife lesion induces glia cells to upregulate GDNF production, which in turn stimulates the axons of the few remaining active dopamine neurons from the substantia nigra and any surrounding dopamine neurons to increase their turnover rate. In addition, GDNF might also help save some of the degenerating 6-OHDA treated neurons. Such neuroprotective effects have been demonstrated in the past [27]. A second possibility is that the lesion severs the processes of the few remaining healthy dopamine neurons from the substantia nigra and any other dopamine neurons in the area, inducing them to grow back and sprout new and more numerous processes. This increase in dopamine would then stimulate the surrounding supporting glia cells to upregulate their production of GDNF. Finally there is the possibility that all of these events are happening independent of one another and are linked only by temporal correlation and not causality.

With the current data it is not possible to favor a single theory. In order to differentiate among the possibilities, further experimentation is needed. A study in which animals would be examined histochemically at more frequent time intervals for additional growth factors and neurotransmitters would establish the temporal expression of such factors indicating the order of up-regulation or down-regulation. In order to establish causality, one must be able to modulate the amount of GDNF and then document the changes. This is currently not possible, but with the advent of knock-down genes it will probably be a future option. In addition, extended studies must be performed to evaluate the long term effects of such treatment and establish whether the behavioral improvement exhibited in this experiment is long lasting. Also, a dose de-escalation study is necessary to determine if the radiation dose that can induce regeneration has to be necrotizing or if non-necrotizing doses of 20 Gy or less can elicit the same effects.

Conclusions

This study demonstrated that Gamma Knife radiosurgery applied to the striatum of hemiparkinsonian rats is effective in promoting GDNF expression resulting in significant improvement of parkinsonian behavior. These changes are believed to represent radiation induced regeneration in the adult mammalian CNS.

References

1. Arenas E, Trupp M, Akerud P, Ibanez CF (1995) GDNF prevents degeneration and promotes the phenotype of brain noradrenergic neurons in vivo. Neuron 15(6): 1465–1473
2. Bankiewicz KS, Plunkett RJ, Jacobowitz DM, Kopin IJ, Oldfield EH (1991) Fetal nondopaminergic neural implants in parkinsonian primates. Histochemical and behavioral studies. J Neurosurg 74(1): 97–104
3. Bankiewicz KS, Plunkett RJ, Jacobowitz DM, Porrino L, di Porzio U, London WT, Kopin IJ, Oldfield EH (1990) The effect of fetal mesencephalon implants on primate MPTP-induced parkinsonism. Histochemical and behavioral studies. J Neurosurg 72(2): 231–244
4. Bankiewicz KS, Plunkett RJ, Kopin IJ, Jacobowitz DM, London WT, Oldfield EH (1988) Transient behavioral recovery in hemiparkinsonian primates after adrenal medullary allografts. Prog Brain Res 78: 543–549
5. Bankiewicz KS, Plunkett RJ, Mefford I, Kopin IJ, Oldfield EH (1990) Behavioral recovery from MPTP-induced parkinsonism in monkeys after intracerebral tissue implants is not related to CSF concentrations of dopamine metabolites. Prog Brain Res 82: 561–571
6. Beck KD, Valverde J, Alexi T, Poulsen K, Moffat B, Vandlen RA, Rosenthal A, Hefti F (1995) Mesencephalic dopaminergic neurons protected by GDNF from axotomy-induced degeneration in the adult brain. Nature 373(6512): 339–341
7. Boer GJ (1994) Ethical guidelines for the use of human embryonic or fetal tissue for experimental and clinical neurotransplantation and research. Network of European CNS Transplantation and Restoration (NECTAR). J Neurol 242(1): 1–13
8. Cass WA (1996) GDNF selectively protects dopamine neurons over serotonin neurons against the neurotoxic effects of methamphetamine. J Neurosci 16(24): 8132–8139
9. Date I, Imaoka T, Miyoshi Y, Ono T, Asari S, Ohmoto T (1996) Chromaffin cell survival and host dopaminergic fiber recovery in a patient with Parkinson's disease treated by cografts of adrenal medulla and pretransected peripheral nerve. Case report. J Neurosurg 84(4): 685–689. review
10. Forno LS, Langston JW (1991) Unfavorable outcome of adrenal medullary transplant for Parkinson's disease. Acta Neuropathol (Berl) 81(6): 691–694
11. Friehs GM, Ojakangas CL, Pachatz P, Schröttner O, Ott E, Pendl G (1995) Thalamotomy and caudatotomy with the Gamma Knife as a treatment for parkinsonism with a comment on lesion sizes. Stereotact Funct Neurosurg 64 [Suppl] 1: 209–221
12. Friehs GM, Ojakangas CL, Schröttner O, Ott E, Pendl G (1997) Radiosurgical lesioning of the caudate nucleus as a treatment for parkinsonism: a preliminary report. Neurol Res 19(1): 97–103
13. Friehs GM, Parker RG, He LS, Haines SJ, Turner DA, Ebner TJ (1991) Lesioning of the striatum reverses motor asymmetry in the 6-hydroxydopamine rodent model of parkinsonism. J Neural Transplant Plast 2(2): 141–156
14. Hoffman AF, van Horne CG, Eken S, Hoffer BJ, Gerhardt GA (1997) In vivo microdialysis studies on somatodendritic dopamine release in the rat substantia nigra: effects of unilateral 6-OHDA lesions and GDNF. Exp Neurol 147(1): 130–141
15. Hudson JL, van Horne CG, Stromberg I, Brock S, Clayton J, Masserano J, Hoffer BJ, Gerhardt GA (1993) Correlation of apomorphine- and amphetamine-induced turning with nigrostriatal dopamine content in unilateral 6-hydroxydopamine lesioned rats. Brain Res 626(1–2): 167–174
16. Jochemsen H (1994) Transplantation of fetal tissue: a medical and ethical assessment, with special attention for the treatment of patients with Parkinson's disease. Ethics Med 10(3): 56–57
17. Kearns CM, Gash DM (1995) GDNF protects nigral dopamine neurons against 6-hydroxydopamine in vivo. Brain Res 672(1–2): 104–111
18. Lin LF, Doherty DH, Lile JD, Bektesh S, Collins F (1993) GDNF: a glial cell line-derived neurotrophic factor for midbrain dopaminergic neurons. Science 260(5111): 1130–1132
19. McCullagh P (1988) Fetal brain transplantation – the scope of the ethical issue. Ethics Med 4(3): 37–39
20. Northoff G (1996) Do brain tissue transplants alter personal identity? Inadequacies of some "standard" arguments. J Med Ethics 22(3): 174–180
21. Palca J (1988) Ethical questions of tissue transplant. Nature 21: 332(6166): 668
22. Peterson DI, Price ML, Small CS (1989) Autopsy findings in a patient who had an adrenal-to-brain transplant for Parkinson's disease. Neurology 39(2 Pt 1): 235–238
23. Plunkett RJ, Bankiewicz KS, Cummins AC, Miletich RS, Schwartz JP, Oldfield EH (1990) Long-term evaluation of hemiparkinsonian monkeys after adrenal autografting or cavitation alone. J Neurosurg 73(6): 918–926
24. Shults CW, Kimber T, Martin D (1996) Intrastriatal injection of GDNF attenuates the effects of 6-hydroxydopamine. Neuroreport 7(2): 627–631
25. Starr PA, Wichmann T, van Horne C, Bakay RA (1999) Intranigral transplantation of fetal substantia nigra allograft in the hemiparkinsonian rhesus monkey. Cell Transplant 8(1): 37–45
26. Turner DA, Kearney W (1993) Scientific and ethical concerns in neural fetal tissue transplantation. Neurosurgery 33(6): 1031–1037. review
27. Tomac A, Lindqvist E, Lin LF, Ogren SO, Young D, Hoffer BJ, Olson L (1995) Protection and repair of the nigrostriatal dopaminergic system by GDNF in vivo. Nature 373(6512): 335–339
28. Waters C, Itabashi HH, Apuzzo ML, Weiner LP (1990) Adrenal to caudate transplantation–postmortem study. Mov Disord 5(3): 248–250

Correspondence: Gerhard M. Friehs, M.D., 100 Butler Drive, Providence, RI 02906, USA.

Author Index

Index of Keywords

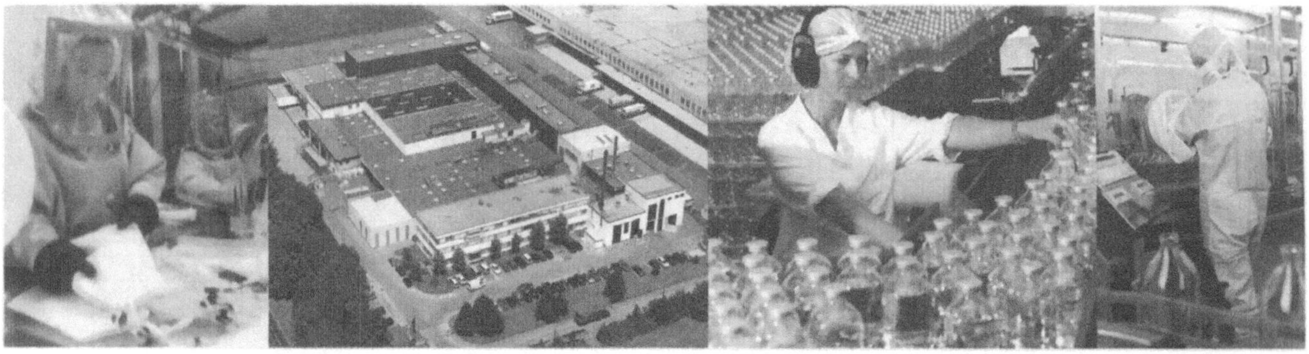

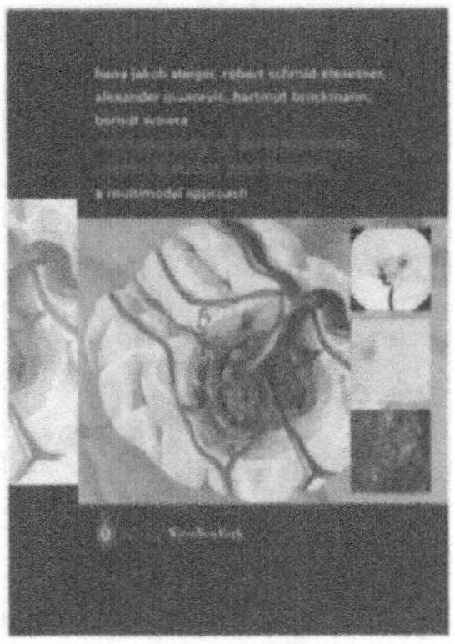

Springer-Verlag
and the Environment

We at Springer-Verlag firmly believe that an international science publisher has a special obligation to the environment, and our corporate policies consistently reflect this conviction.

We also expect our business partners – printers, paper mills, packaging manufacturers, etc. – to commit themselves to using environmentally friendly materials and production processes.

The paper in this book is made from no-chlorine pulp and is acid free, in conformance with international standards for paper permanency.

GPSR Compliance

The European Union's (EU) General Product Safety Regulation (GPSR) is a set of rules that requires consumer products to be safe and our obligations to ensure this.

If you have any concerns about our products, you can contact us on ProductSafety@springernature.com

In case Publisher is established outside the EU, the EU authorized representative is:

Springer Nature Customer Service Center GmbH
Europaplatz 3
69115 Heidelberg, Germany

Batch number: 10731490

Printed by Printforce, the Netherlands